DIRECT REFERRAL SYSTEMS FOR HEARING AID PROVISION

UNIVERSITY OF MANCHESTER

**HESTER ADRIAN
RESEARCH CENTRE**

London: HMSO

ISBN 0 11 321692 0

Acknowledgements

This book is based on research which was funded by the Department of Health. However, the views expressed in it are those of the authors, and are not necessarily the official views of the Department.

A very large number of people have contributed in one way or another to the research reported herein. We would like to thank the original Working Group, which did some considerable spadework before we were even involved, and the subsequent Advisory Group which gave very valuable help throughout the project. Then there are the large number of hard-working Audiological Technicians and Scientists, and ENT Consultants and Doctors, who gave of their time both to be involved in the research and to answer our questions. We also thank the patients who allowed us to interview them, and who made additional trips to the Centres for the ENT Specialist examinations.

We owe a special debt to a few individuals whose contribution was particularly notable. These include Dr Dai Stephens, of the Welsh Hearing Institute, who gave invaluable input concerning audiological matters at all stages of the research; Mr Ken Wright of the Centre for Health Economics at York, who advised on the analysis of costs; and Mr John Schofield FRCS and Mr Charles Smith FRCS, the Consultant ENT Surgeons who made medical examinations of samples of patients for us. Our greatest thanks, however, have to go to the project managers and their teams at the twelve pilot Centres. They not only set up and operated the pilot DR schemes, but somehow managed to also cope with our exorbitant demands regarding form-filling and other data collection. We only hope that the result proves their efforts to have been worthwhile.

David Reeves
Linda Mason
Helen Prosser
Chris Kiernan

The Authors

David Reeves is Research Fellow and Departmental Statistician at the Hester Adrian Research Centre, University of Manchester.

Linda Mason was Research Associate at the Hester Adrian Research Centre, and is now Research Officer at the Public Health Research and Resource Centre, Salford, near Manchester.

Helen Prosser is Research Associate at the Hester Adrian Research Centre, University of Manchester.

Chris Kiernan is Director of the Hester Adrian Research Centre, University of Manchester.

Contents

Part III: Summary of Main Findings

Part I

Department of Health Direct Referral Pilot Projects

David Reeves
Helen Prosser
Linda Mason
Chris Kiernan

1 Introduction

1.1 Background to the research

1.1.1 On 27th July 1989 Mr Roger Freeman, then Parliamentary Under Secretary of State for Health, announced a number of proposals for improving hearing aid services. A major part of Mr Freeman's proposals concerned a plan to speed up the procedure for hearing aid provision:

> '....I have asked my officials with the help of appropriate outside expert advice to draw up and consult interested bodies on a programme of action commencing in the new financial year to expand the number of Direct Referral schemes and set up a mechanism to evaluate them to ensure that they are operating with appropriate safeguards and are effective in reducing waiting times.' (Hansard Written Answers 27 July 1989).

1.1.2 Following the statement, a Working Group was set up to carry forward Mr Freeman's proposals. This led the Department of Health to commission the Hester Adrian Research Centre, in mid-1990, to evaluate Direct Referral procedures.

1.1.3 A total of £558,000 was allocated from the Department's centrally reserved health authority funds to meet the expenditure incurred in setting up and running each of the selected local projects and to cover the cost of evaluating the whole project. The funding provided to the projects was £225,000 in 1990–91 and £247,000 in 1991–92. The amount allocated in the second year took into account factors that had arisen as individual projects developed. The Hester Adrian Research Centre received £86,000 to meet the costs of evaluation.

1.2 Traditional Referral and Direct Referral

1.2.1 Flow diagrams illustrating the Traditional Referral (TR) and Direct Referral (DR) systems of hearing aid provision appear in figure 1.1.

1.2.2 Under the traditional system, GPs refer patients to a hospital-based ENT consultant or audiological physician. The patient receives an ENT examination as a check for the presence of pathology, and normally on the same day the hospital Audiological Unit (or 'Hearing Aid Centre') will conduct audiological tests to assess the hearing loss and will make an impression of the ear or ears. The impression is sent away to have an earmould made from it. When this returns, the patient is recalled, fitted with the hearing aid, and instructed in its use. The great majority of Hearing Aid

Figure 1.1 Flow diagrams showing principal routes of hearing aid provision followed by Traditionally and Directly Referred patients

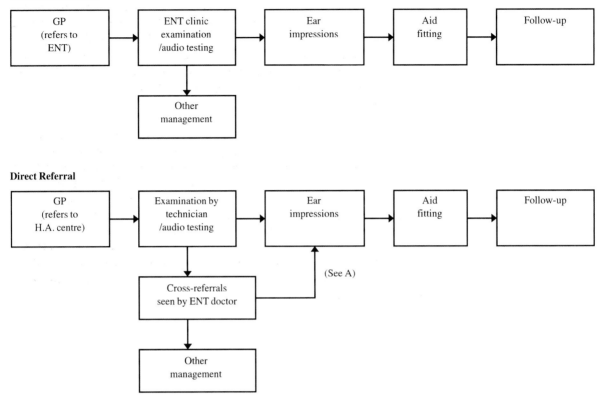

Traditional Referral

GP (refers to ENT) → ENT clinic examination /audio testing → Ear impressions → Aid fitting → Follow-up

ENT clinic examination /audio testing → Other management

Direct Referral

GP (refers to H.A. centre) → Examination by technician /audio testing → Ear impressions → Aid fitting → Follow-up

Examination by technician /audio testing → Cross-referrals seen by ENT doctor → (See A) → Ear impressions

Cross-referrals seen by ENT doctor → Other management

A) A substantial proportion of cross-referrals have the ear impressions, and sometimes fitting, before seeing the ENT doctor

Centres will recall the patient again in one to three months time in order to review their progress. In addition, some patients may be referred on to a hearing therapist or social worker. Environmental aids (e.g. special doorbells) or commercial hearing aids may be dispensed in certain circumstances.

1.2.3 The Direct Referral procedure is exactly the same as the above, except that GPs instead refer appropriate patients directly to the Hearing Aid Centre. GPs are expected to ensure that such patients show no signs of significant ear abnormalities. An audiological technician examines the patients (using a set of guidelines) for potential medical conditions. Those who fail are cross-referred to the ENT department.

1.2.4 The traditional system is under great pressure in this country. This often results in long delays between a patient being referred by their GP and being seen by an ENT doctor. The delay can sometimes be as long as two years (RNID 1984). The Working Group set up to carry Mr Freeman's statement forward conducted a short postal survey of health authorities. Of 74 that replied, 25% reported average waiting times for an ENT examination of six months or longer. In three authorities the average wait was a year or more. There would then be a further delay before the aid was fitted.

1.2.5 The primary aim of DR schemes is to reduce waiting times by removing a significant proportion of patients from ENT waiting lists, thus speeding up the process both for them and for those in the ENT queue. The Royal National Institute for the Deaf in their publication 'Hearing Aids – the Case for Change' (1988), recommended the adoption of DR procedures. They also wanted to see a new professional group created, 'Community Dispensers', who would be responsible for DR patients.

1.2.6 A high proportion of health authorities have already experimented with DR schemes. One aspect of the present research was a national survey of Hearing Aid Centres. This found that 39% operate or had operated DR systems (the survey is discussed in Part II of this report). While many of these schemes appear to have been successful in reducing waiting times, prior to the present study there had been little attempt to evaluate this rigorously. Furthermore, the DR procedure raises many other issues which need to be properly addressed. Principal amongst these is the matter of safety, as there is considerable concern that the procedure may miss some cases of significant pathology. Other important issues include patient and staff satisfaction and the cost of the procedure.

2 Methodology

2.1 Aims of the research

2.1.1 Mr Freeman's statement (section 1.1) contained two key elements. One was to expand the number of DR schemes, and the other was to evaluate Direct Referral. The evaluation of Direct Referral procedures necessarily had to involve some degree of comparison with the traditional referral system. To meet the twin requirements, a research program with two major strands was implemented. The first of these was the setting up of a number of 'pilot' DR schemes at Hearing Aid Centres in different health authorities. Each of these schemes was to run for a full year. The schemes were evaluated while they were in operation, with additional evaluations of the TR procedure at these Centres both immediately prior to the start of DR, and again towards the end of the pilot period.

2.1.2 The second research strand was a national survey to identify those DR schemes already in existence, followed by interviewing at a selected number of these. This exercise was sufficiently large and different to warrant a report of its own. This appears as 'Part II' of this volume. However, some references to the results are made in Part I, where appropriate.

2.2 Selection of health authorities

2.2.1 In February 1990 all district health authorities in England were asked by means of a letter if they would be interested in bidding for funds to set up a Direct Referral scheme which would run for one year and be subject to evaluation.

2.2.2 From the returns, twenty-one DHAs who at that time did not operate Direct Referral were selected and asked to put in a bid. These were not selected to be a representative sample: rather, they satisfied certain criteria concerning waiting times, patient volume, geographical spacing, and so on. One of the concerns was to ensure that a good variety of types were included, including large and small Centres, a range of waiting times and patient volumes, and rural and urban environments. However, Centres with very minimal waiting times and/or patient volumes were excluded.

2.2.3 A total of fifteen bids were received, and twelve Centres were selected who received finance to establish a DR system and take part in the evaluation.

2.2.4 The setting up of the DR schemes was largely the responsibility of Centres themselves. However, they were required to follow certain guide-lines and conditions laid down by the evaluators in order to ensure as much compatibility as possible across the twelve projects for the purposes of evaluation.

2.2.5 One important prerequisite for inclusion as a pilot Centre was that all patients going through the DR route must receive a 'safety-check' by an ENT doctor. This requirement was necessary to ensure that standards of patient safety were maintained during the pilot period. It also formed an essential element of the evaluation of the safety of Direct Referral.

2.3 Aims of the evaluation

2.3.1 The evaluation was designed with a number of principal areas of interest in mind. These were:
1) WAITING TIMES. The principal advantage of Direct Referral schemes was expected to be that they reduce the time it takes for a patient, having been referred by a GP, to be fitted with a hearing aid. Assessing this was one of the major aims of the research.
2) SAFETY. Direct Referral, by removing the ENT examination, relies upon either the GP or the audiological technician to screen out those patients who need to be seen in the ENT department. There is concern that some patients with medical conditions may fail to be identified, and therefore not receive the appropriate management. The safety of the procedure was therefore a crucial consideration.
3) QUALITY ASSURANCE. There needs to be assurance that, at the very least, the quality of service to patients is not reduced under DR. Waiting times and safety are obviously vital elements of quality assurance, but there are others which also needed evaluation, including patient satisfaction, queuing times (in waiting rooms), number of appointments required, and time spent on appointments.
4) STAFF SATISFACTION. The satisfaction of both technical and ENT staff with the schemes needed to be assessed.
5) COST EFFECTIVENESS. The cost of DR compared to TR was an important consideration. Any cost differences then needed to be looked at in the light of the pros and cons of the two systems.

In addition to the above, the opportunity was taken to examine a substantial number of other important, but less central, issues.

2.4 Research design

2.4.1 In discussing the research design, the point first needs to be made that when DR is introduced TR does not come to an end, but rather the two systems operate in parallel. Not all hearing aid patients are suitable for DR, as a proportion will always have additional factors that need to be seen by an ENT doctor prior to hearing aid assessment and fitting – if only to have them passed as non-significant. Part of a normal DR system is that GPs are expected to select only appropriate patients for Direct Referral, sending others via the traditional route. Usually, the hospital ENT surgeons provide

GPs with a set of guidelines to aid them in selecting appropriate patients. This was the case at all but one of the pilot projects (see 4.3.2).

2.4.2 The methodology of evaluation centred upon using each Centre as its own control. A first phase of data collection was undertaken when each service was exclusively TR, before the Direct Referral system was introduced. During the pilot period, data on DR patients was collected on an ongoing fashion as they passed through the provision process. Then in the last few months of the pilots a second phase of information gathering on the TR procedure was undertaken, plus some further data collection on DR patients.

2.4.3 The design was intended to allow two principal types of comparison to be made. The first was a comparison of TR prior to the pilot schemes with DR during the pilot period. The second was a comparison of some aspects of TR – most notably waiting times – prior to DR with the same aspects of TR towards the end of the pilots.

2.4.4 In addition to the above, a further element had to be built into the design concerned with evaluating the safety of the DR procedures. All DR patients seen by technicians during the pilot period also received a safety-check examination by an ENT doctor. The results of these examinations allowed an assessment to be made of how many cases of significant pathology were missed by technicians, what the pathologies were, and how serious.

2.4.5 It is possible, however, that there are cases of missed pathology amongst patients served via the TR system. For a full evaluation the rate of failure under DR needed to be compared to the rate under TR. In order to do this, two 'External Specialists' were employed to conduct examinations of samples of TR and DR patients at a number of the pilot Centres. At each Centre the TR and DR samples were seen by the same specialist, who was 'blind' to the route taken by each patient. This ensured that the computed failure rates would be directly comparable.

3 Summary of Data Collected

3.1 Introduction

3.1.1 Subsequent chapters are organised according to various topics of interest. In examining and discussing any one of these, use may be made of results drawn from more than one of the various sets of data that were collected. Consequently, it has been found convenient to present the details of all the data-sets in this single section prior to the presentation of any analysis. The evaluation entailed collection of a broad range of information from a variety of data sources. A schematic diagram illustrating the principal sets of data collected appears in figure 3.1. The sample sizes are summarized in table 3.1.

Table 3.1
Summary of sample sizes

	TR patients interviews	DR patients interviews	Pro-formas on TRs fitted prior to pilot	Pro-formas on TRs fitted during pilot	Pro-formas on DR patients
Orange	20	2	99	71	50 and 105*
Red	19	17	99	94	106
Yellow	20	21	94	54	247
Green	21	14	100	74	190
Blue	19	27	97	81	652
White	19	19	97	64	398
Black	0	22	0	66	186
Grey	21	19	54	0	181
Brown	20	20	95	100	304
Silver	22	21	100	45	312
Gold	20	18	99	98	266
Bronze	20	22	97	54	185
Total	221	222	1031	801	3132

*Orange completed 50 Patient Details sheets, but 105 Technician Examination sheets.

3.1.2 For the purposes of presenting results, all of the Centres have been given code names, consisting of the names of colours (e.g. Yellow, Black), and all text and tables refer to the Centres solely by these codes. This is to maintain confidentiality with respect to the findings for individual Centres.

Figure 3.1
Schematic diagram of data
collected on pilot schemes

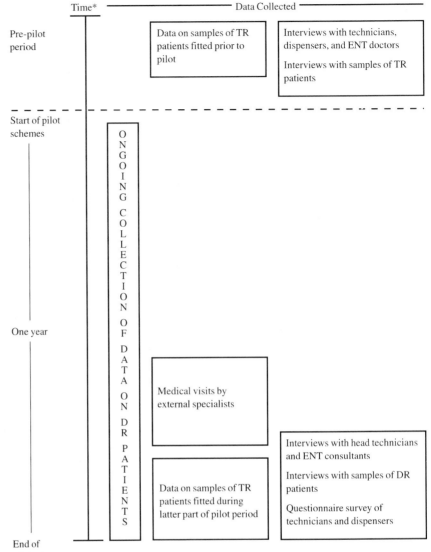

*The time-line is only approximate: specific times differed between projects

3.2 Interviews with staff

3.2.1 There were two interview periods at each of the 12 projects. The first shortly before DR began, the second during the last months of each project.

3.2.2 In the first period, interviews were conducted with as many of the audiological technicians and private dispensers who would be involved in examining DR patients as possible, and also with as many ENT doctors as made themselves available. Interviews were conducted with a total of 35 NHS technicians, 4 private dispensers, and 39 ENT doctors.

3.2.3 The purpose of these interviews was to obtain, firstly, some background to each of the projects, including such things as the reasons for wanting to implement DR, details of the current service, and intentions with respect to the operation of the schemes. Secondly, to ascertain what each group (technicians and doctors) saw as the important issues in the hearing aid service.

3.2.4 The interviews were semi-structured and to a large degree exploratory, being intended, as they were, to identify salient issues. Consequently, these pre-pilot interviews are not discussed further in this report, though much of the factual data they produced is reported. Their importance lies instead in the fact that they were the main source from which the structured interview schedules used in the pre-existing schemes, and those used in the second round of interviewing at the pilot projects, were derived.

3.2.5 It proved to be not practical to try and interview the same set of individuals in the second round of interviews towards the end of the pilot period. In the event, some had had little or no involvement in the projects, while others who had not been interviewed were in some instances heavily involved. Therefore, the second round of interviews focused on three groups: a) the head technicians; b) one consultant from each Centre who had good knowledge of the pilot and its effects from an ENT point of view; c) at least one other ENT doctor from each Centre who had conducted a high proportion of safety-checks. In all, interviews with head technicians were conducted at all 12 Centres, interviews with consultants were done at 10 (this could not be arranged at the other two), and 15 other interviews were done with safety-check doctors. The interviews concentrated on staff opinions regarding the success or otherwise of the project, any problems encountered, and the perceived benefits and disadvantages of the schemes.

3.3 Interviews with patients

3.3.1 Interviews were conducted with TR patients prior to the start of DR, and with DR patients fitted towards the end of each project. The aim was to interview 20 TR patients and 20 DR patients at each Centre. The interview schedules were very much the same for both sets of patients. The information collected covered such items as details of the appointments attended, satisfaction with the service received, times spent travelling to appointments and queuing to be seen, etc.

3.3.2 There was only a short time between the commissioning of the research and implementation of the DR schemes, and the interviews with TR patients had to be conducted in this period. Consequently, there was no time for a formal piloting of the questionnaire. Instead, amendments were made following the first couple of interview sessions. As a result, for the first two Centres visited, Orange and Blue, there is some missing data on one or two questions which were added later.

3.3.3 The original intention was to interview patients when they came back for a review, one to three months (depending on the Centre) after fitting.

This was so that satisfaction with the hearing aid itself, and other issues related to rehabilitation, could be assessed. However, the first few interview sessions quickly demonstrated that this strategy was not working. The biggest problem was that only around 50% of patients were turning up for the review. This was doubling the number of visits needed to collect data, and, it was felt, making the sample unrepresentative: patients who lived furthest from the Centre, those who were disabled, and those who had given up with the aid altogether, were less likely to return for review. Also, it was apparent that the time-span since fitting was not sufficient to say very much about rehabilitation, as many patients had not even got used to using the aid properly yet. Finally, nearly all patients were elderly and many had memory difficulties, and waiting until the review before interviewing was reducing the reliability of the information they could give concerning previous appointments.

3.3.4 As a result of all these difficulties, after the first few interview sessions interviewing at review was abandoned, along with the attempt to assess satisfaction with the aid and other rehabilitation issues. All subsequent interviews of TR patients, and all interviews of DR patients, were done at the fitting appointment (with just the occasional exception). This was far more successful, as nearly all patients turned up for the fitting, the information collected about that appointment was precise, and information concerning previous appointments was more reliable.

3.3.5 With regard to the interviews with TR patients, due to time pressure one Centre (Black) was excluded from this exercise. A total of 221 interviews with TR patients were conducted across the other 11 Centres.

3.3.6 Interviews with DR patients were conducted during the last half of each project. Each scheme was given at least 6 months to 'settle in' before any interviewing of DR patients was undertaken. Again, the target was 20 patient interviews at each Centre. However, at some Centres the rate of referrals was low and, despite multiple interview visits, it proved difficult to achieve the target. Consequently, in some places a fairly severe shortfall had to be accepted. At one Centre, Orange, it was not possible to arrange dates on which to interview patients despite a large number of attempts. Only 2 were achieved, and therefore no results for DR interviews at this site are presented. Overall, a total of 222 DR patient interviews were conducted.

3.4 Questionnaire survey of technicians and dispensers

3.4.1 Towards the end of each project the technicians and private dispensers who had examined Direct Referral patients during the pilot were provided with a structured questionnaire to complete and return. Head technicians were excepted from this, as they were interviewed directly. The exercise was done such that the replies were kept confidential from other staff at each Centre. The questionnaire covered the impact of DR on the technician's/dispenser's job, problems encountered, opinions about the scheme, and a number of other issues. Returns were received from 26 technicians and 3 dispensers.

3.5 Data on samples of TR patients

3.5.1 Each project was asked to provide data on two samples of 100 TR patients. The first was 100 TR patients fitted shortly before the start of DR; the second was 100 TR patients fitted in the latter part of the project period. In order to maximise comparability with patients seen under DR, these samples were restricted to patients within the same age-range as the age criteria for Direct Referral.

3.5.2 The reason for collecting these samples was: firstly, to obtain data on the TR service prior to DR, including waiting times, the grades of doctors seeing TR patients, types of aids fitted, and so on; and secondly to determine how the service to TR patients had changed over the course of the DR pilot, particularly with regards to waiting times.

3.5.3 Most Centres reached the target of 100 patients for the first sample, or came very close to it, by drawing the information from hospital notes. At Black, TR patients had the impressions and fitting at a different hospital to the pilot Centre, and because of the complexity of getting patient records from the second hospital this Centre was excluded from the exercise. All in all, completed forms were received for a total of 1031 TR patients fitted prior to DR.

3.5.4 The second sample was generally collected as patients passed through the provision process, as this was less time-consuming than recalling hospital notes and taking the information from those. Because of referral rates, work-load, and time constraints, many Centres could not reach the target of 100, and one Centre, Grey, did not provide a second sample.

3.5.5 In the event, the shortfall has not proved serious, because the pre-DR sample has proved to be the most important, in terms of comparing the two systems, and the second sample has been large enough for analysis purposes. In all, forms were returned for 801 TR patients fitted during the latter part of the projects.

3.6 Data collection on DR patients

3.6.1 Projects were required to record data on each DR patient as he/she travelled through the process of provision. Due to time constraints, it was not possible to continue the data collection up to the review appointment, and therefore the appointment for fitting was taken as the end-point of data collection.

3.6.2 The Centres were asked to complete three data collection forms for each DR patient they saw. These forms were supplied by the evaluators. The first was for recording details of the patient, and for each procedure undertaken (audio testing, impression taking, and fitting) the date, who did it, how much time it took, and so on. The second form was for details of the technician's examination of the patient, and the actions decided on. The third form was completed by the ENT doctor at the time of the safety-check, and again was for recording the details of the examination and the actions required. The pro-formas appear in appendix I.I.

3.6.3 At 10 Centres there was little or no difficulty with this aspect of the data-collection (at least from the evaluators point of view – many Centres found it an onerous task). At Orange, however, a number of problems were encountered. None of the first or third forms were completed, and the second form was only kept for a minority of patients. Consequently, data on DR patients at this Centre is very partial. In particular, there is no information on the findings of the ENT safety-checks, and the Centre has had to be excluded from analyses which draw on this. Fortunately, after the project the head technician completed the first form for a sample of 50 DR patients seen towards the end of the project, so there is some limited information on patient details and the appointments kept.

3.6.4 The other Centre where there were problems was Red. This Centre had designed their own Technician Examination Form prior to the project and wished to use it, particularly as they had set up a corresponding computer data-entry program. Unfortunately, the form did not record whether a patient was cross-referred to ENT or not. It will be seen in later sections that information about cross-referral is an important element in some analyses, and in consequence this Centre has sometimes had to be excluded.

3.6.5 The numbers of DR patients for whom forms were returned varies considerably. The smallest numbers were 105 from Orange and 106 from Red. The largest were 652 from Blue, and 398 from White. Overall, pro-formas were received for a total of 3132 DR patients.

3.6.6 It should be noted that this does not represent all patients directly referred during the pilot period. Some Centres did not return forms for particularly inappropriate referrals (e.g. patients who were found to already possess NHS hearing aids, those under the criteria age-limit), and a number of patients never turned up at the Centres. Also, there were probably a number of other cases for which – for one reason or another – forms were not completed or returned.

3.6.7 In a number of cases information was missing on some data-items, and because of this sample sizes vary somewhat from one analysis to another. In particular, the sheet recording details of the technician examination was missing for 90 cases, and the ENT examination sheet was missing for 668. Nearly two-thirds of this latter figure is accounted for by just three Centres: Orange, which completed no ENT sheets; Silver, where a large proportion of patients had not yet received safety-checks when data-collection ended; and the private dispenser scheme at Blue, where a large proportion never attended the safety-check. Missing sheets at other Centres were principally due to non-attendance.

3.7 Medical visits by External Specialists

3.7.1 Two 'External Specialists' were employed to visit a number of the Centres and make independent ENT examinations of samples of TR and DR patients. The evaluators were fortunate to obtain the services of Mr Charles Smith (FRCS) of York and Mr John Schofield (FRCS) of Warwick. Both are individuals of high standing in the field. Mr Smith is President of the European Federation of Otolaryngology Society Members, and an ex-President of the British Association of Otolaryngologists. Mr Schofield is a past President of the Midland Institute of Otolaryngology and a past President of the Laryngology Section of the Royal Society of Medicine. He was also chairman of the British Academic Conference in Otolaryngology, an international conference. Both have published in the field.

3.7.2 The specialists between them visited nine of the 12 Centres. Three schemes, at Grey, Black, and Silver, were excluded from this exercise, principally on the grounds that they did not have sufficient staff or space to carry it through. One other Centre, Brown, was initially excluded but later included because of the involvement of a private dispenser there. One specialist visited four 'Northern' Centres, and the other five 'Southern' Centres. They used a pro-forma similar to that used by the local ENT doctors doing safety-checks, but requiring more detail in those cases where they felt that some form of further investigation or intervention was needed. This appears in appendix I.II. The visits were made towards the end of each project, between September 1991 and January 1992.

3.7.3 The original aim was that 30 TR and 30 DR patients would be examined in each Centre – with the exception of Brown, where the aim was 15 of each. This would yield totals of 255 TRs and 255 DRs. In the event, due to patient non-attendance there was some shortfall on the target figure in every Centre. The actual totals examined were 216 TR patients and 239 DR patients. More details on the methodology of the external specialist visits are given in section 10.2.

3.8 Service statistics

3.8.1 An attempt was made to collect some service statistics from each Centre, principally to judge whether the introduction of DR affected demand at all. It was discovered early on that levels of statistical collection vary widely from place to place: some Hearing Aid Centres produce no routine statistics at all, while others generate a wide range of statistical measures. At the end of the day, the only measure that was consistently available from most Centres was the numbers of hearing aids fitted. Where possible, figures for these were obtained on a monthly basis for the project period and on a yearly basis for up to three years preceding.

4 Characteristics of the Pilot Centres and Direct Referral Schemes

4.1 Background characteristics

4.1.1 Table 4.1 summarizes the principal background variables characterizing each Centre. It should be noted that the figures in this table are mainly what Centres reported prior to the project, and in some instances are of doubtful accuracy. These were, however, the basis upon which Centres were selected to be participants in the study. The only figures that have been checked and corrected where necessary are those pertaining to staff numbers.

4.1.2 The Centres were spread throughout England, all the way from the Southwest and Southeast to the Northwest and Northeast. Seven Centres served predominantly urban populations, while five were principally rural, and the size of the populations served varied between 175,000 and 900,000. The Centres were very variable in terms of numbers of staff: the single largest Centre had 8 ENT consultants, 11 other ENT doctors, 2 audiological scientists, and 9 technicians; the smallest had 1 consultant, 3 other ENT doctors, and just 2.5 technicians. Numbers of new patients fitted with hearing aids correspond to some degree with Centre size, but not entirely. The smallest number was 500 fittings per annum, and the largest 3000.

4.1.3 With regard to the number of weeks wait between GP referral and aid fitting, a range is given in some cases. This is where there were different waits at different community sites, or where the wait for special ENT 'hearing aid clinics' (where a number of patients referred for a hearing aid are seen in one go) differed from those for normal ENT clinics. Three Centres reported relatively short waiting times, of 4 months or less. In contrast, at three others the expected wait – for at least some groups of patients – was over 1 year, and at another two it was only a little short of this.

4.2 Special features of the projects
(table 4.2)

4.2.1 In the main, the DR pilot projects were of a fairly standard form, with GPs being asked to refer appropriate patients direct to a main Hearing Aid Centre, where they would be examined and assessed for a hearing aid by a senior NHS audiological technician. The technician would cross-refer to ENT any patients he or she considered needed more management than just the fitting of a hearing aid. Occasionally a patient would be referred back to their GP or elsewhere (e.g. Hearing Therapy) if the technician deemed it appropriate.

Table 4.1 Background details of each pilot centre

	Type of area	Population served	Number of GPs in area	New fittings per annum	ENT Cons	Other ENT doctors	Aud. Scientists	Technicians	Hearing Therapists	Wait (weeks) GP to fit
A	Rural	407,000	237	1016	3	5	1	4	2	60
B	Urban	320,000	170	500	3	7.5	1	2	2	16
C	Urban	650,000	Unknown	3000	4	8	1.5	7	0	29–87
D	Rural	900,000	465	2472	6	8	0	2	2	42
E	Urban	324,000	167	1284	3	6	0	4	0.5	19–21
F	Urban	452,000	216	950	3	6	3	5	2	26–34
G	Rural	169,000	91	680	1	3	0	2.5	0	35–53
H	Urban	Unknown	Unknown	1496	8	11	2	9	0	14
I	Rural	302,000	180	1075	2	4	0	3	0	45
J	Rural	175,000	91	900	2	3	0	4	0	26
K	Urban	365,000	420	700	2	5	2	4	0	19–59
L	Urban	262,000	317	750	1.4	3	0	6	0	8–14

Note: To preserve the identity of the Centres involved code names have been removed and the row order randomized.

Table 4.2 Special features of the pilot schemes

	Involvement of private sector	All or part community based	Age-limit for DR patients	Other unusual features
Orange	No	No	18 Years	
Red	No	No	60	Selected patients for DR from GP letters to ENT. Operating waiting list initiative at time of start of pilot.
Yellow	Yes	Yes	18	Transferred TR patients across to DR scheme. Technicians dewaxed DR patients.
Green	No	No	60	
Blue	Yes	Yes	60	
White	No	Yes	55	
Black	No	No	18	Did no fittings of TR patients.
Grey	Yes	Yes	25	Technical staff numbers reduced shortly before pilot, greatly disrupting TR service.
Brown	Yes	Yes	18	
Silver	No	No	60	
Gold	No	Yes	60	
Bronze	No	No	18 Years	

4.2.2 There were two further elements however, which Centres that bid for funding were asked to consider building into their schemes. These were the involvement of the private sector, and community provision outside of the main hospital base.

4.2.3 Four Centres involved the private sector in some fashion: Yellow, Blue, Grey, and Brown. At Yellow and Brown, private dispensers (one at each) were employed who worked alongside the NHS technicians doing exactly the same job. The situations at both Blue and Grey were rather different, and because they have implications for the understanding of subsequent sections of the report, it is important that they be explained at this point.

4.2.4 At Blue, a private dispenser was involved who ran his own 'sub-scheme' at community sites largely independent of the NHS project. Referrals would come in to the main NHS hospital, and be shared out on a 'one-to-one' basis between the NHS project and the dispenser. After this, the dispenser would make his own appointments with the patients, and manage them independently of the NHS. In view of this arrangement, it has been found convenient to regard the NHS and dispenser schemes at Blue as being in effect two separate projects, and they are treated thus in subsequent sections and in most tables, where they are referred to as 'BLUE(NH)' and 'BLUE(PD)'.

4.2.5 The private sector involvement at Grey was different again. The scheme there began with all DR patients being seen at community sites by a dispenser who was an employee of a private company. Half-way through the project, however, this arrangement collapsed, and – after a pause – the scheme was taken over by the inhouse NHS technicians, who ran it for the remaining period. For this Centre, therefore, results for the first half of the pilot relate to the dispenser, and those for the second half to the NHS technicians.

4.2.6 At six Centres at least part of the DR service was located in the community. This aspect of the projects is dealt with in detail in a later section, and so will not be discussed further at this point.

4.2.7 One other important feature of the projects which differed was the age-limit for DR patients. The great majority of candidates for hearing aids are over 60 years of age. Most cases of loss over this age are usually regarded as being due to irreversible or non-dangerous factors. Conversely, significant hearing loss at a younger age has a good probability of being due to serious or remediable conditions. Consequently, the vast majority of DR schemes in existence do not accept patients below 60, or in some cases 65 or 70. However, under the pilot schemes all DR patients received an ENT safety-examination, and therefore the working group felt that Centres should be given the opportunity to accept patients of a lower age, if they felt it appropriate. In the event, five Centres set the limit at 60 years, one at 55 years, one at 25 years, and five at 18 years.

4.3 Other non-standard features

4.3.1 Three of the projects exhibited other non-standard features in addition to the above.

4.3.2 *Red*. This Centre did not ask GPs themselves to choose patients for DR, but instead selected patients referred to ENT where the GP's letter indicated that the patient was over 60 years old, had no symptom other than hearing difficulty, and only required a hearing aid. Staff at Red had developed a fairly complex experimental design which they wished to implement, of which this was a part.

4.3.3 *Yellow*. This Centre transferred patients who had been waiting a long time in the TR queue across to the DR system. This was against instructions given to Centres prior to the start. When questioned about this, the Centre replied that they had felt it unethical to leave these patients in the (very long) ENT queue while new patients were being seen quickly. This was also the only Centre where technicians undertook dewaxing of patients.

4.3.4 *Black*. Here, the provision service prior to the project was split across two hospitals. TR patients had the ENT examination and audiometric testing at Black, but had to go to another hospital (which controlled the hearing aid budget) for ear impressions and fitting of the aid. Subsequent reviews, however, were done at Black. During the pilot, the whole of the provision process for DR patients was at Black, but TR patients continued under the old system.

5 Characteristics of DR and TR Patients

5.1 Sex
(table 5.1)

5.1.1 At most Centres, female DR patients slightly outnumbered males, with the proportion of females typically being around 55–60%. In only one Centre, Orange, was there more males (55%), while at two others, Blue(PD) and Grey, the balance was more-or-less even. The comparative figures for TR patients show a more-or-less identical picture.

Table 5.1
Sex distribution (figures in percentages)

| | Traditional Referral | | Direct Referral | | Sample size | |
	male	female	male	female	TR	DR
Orange	58%	42%	55%	45%	99	49
Red	40	60	43	57	99	106
Yellow	32	68	41	59	95	247
Green	42	58	38	62	100	190
Blue(NH)	43	57	41	59	100	277
Blue(PD)	not applicable		48	52	na	374
White	43	57	39	61	97	378
Black	46*	54*	41	59	66*	173
Grey	52	48	51	49	54	176
Brown	49	51	47	53	97	283
Silver	50	50	39	61	100	307
Gold	42	58	43	57	100	266
Bronze	44	56	42	58	97	172

*Figures for Black based on TR patients seen during pilot, all others based on pre-pilot TR sample.

5.2 Age
(table 5.2)

5.2.1 It will be seen from the table that some Centres which adopted a sixty-years plus age criteria, in fact saw a small number of patients below this age. These were patients close to the age-limit who were referred.

5.2.2 The five Centres that took DRs from age 18 years, in the main received very few referrals of under sixty. The highest proportion of under-sixties was 13%, at Brown, and the next highest was 9%, at Bronze. All of these Centres could have imposed a minimum age of 60 years with only a small effect on the total number of referrals received. In all but two Centres quite a substantial proportion of DR patients were eighty or over, typically 35–45% of the total. The exceptions to this were Orange (20%, but based on a small sample) and Red (26%). It is not known whether this reflects demographic features of these areas.

Table 5.2 Age distributions (figures in percentages)

Note: TR sample restricted to same age-range as DR patients.

	DR age criteria	Traditional Referrals				Direct Referrals				Sample size	
		<60	60–69	70–79	80+	<60	60–69	70–79	80+	TR	DR
Orange	18	21%	23%	40%	15%	–	27%	53%	20%	99	49
Red	60	–	30	42	27	0	32	42	26	99	103
Yellow	18	3	15	36	46	3	17	45	35	94	245
Green	60	–	24	49	27	2	24	35	40	100	190
Blue(NH)	60	–	20	40	40	<1	16	40	42	97	267
Blue(PD)	60		not applicable			<1	22	40	39	na	371
White	55	4	15	50	31	3	16	40	41	97	376
Black	18	11*	20*	42*	27*	4	15	36	44	66*	169
Grey	25	17	26	33	24	7	17	36	40	54	168
Brown	18	16	16	39	30	13	16	35	36	95	278
Silver	60	–	16	49	35	<1	16	46	38	100	304
Gold	60	–	27	40	32	2	25	40	34	99	266
Bronze	18	13	21	34	32	9	15	38	38	97	163

*Figures for Black based on TR patients seen during pilot, all others based on pre-pilot TR sample.

5.3 Aid fitted
(table 5.3)

5.3.1 By far the most common aids fitted to DR patients were Series 10 aids. These accounted for a minimum of 68% of fittings at Yellow, up to a maximum of 97% at Blue(PD). Most of the remaining fittings were Series 30, with just a smattering of fittings of Series 50, bodyworn, and private aids. Regarding the latter, a total of just 4 private aids were fitted, with 3 of these being at the same Centre, Silver.

Table 5.3 Types of aids fitted (figures in percentages)

Note: 10=series 10; 30=series 30; 50=series 50; BW=bodyworn; COMM=commercial

	Traditional Referrals					Direct Referrals					2nd TR sample series 10	Sample size		
	10	30	50	BW	COMM	10	30	50	BW	COMM		TR	DR	2nd TR
Orange	80%	18%	2%	–	–	83%	17%	–	–	–	84%	97	49	69
Red	76	24	–	–	–	81	16	3	–	–	66	97	98	94
Yellow	62	32	5	1	–	68	31	<1	–	–	65	95	227	49
Green	71	27	2	–	–	92	8	–	–	–	86	100	154	70
Blue(NH)	83	14	1	1	1	95	4	<1	–	–	90	100	261	81
Blue(PD)		not applicable				97	1	–	1	–	na	na	350	na
White	73	23	3	1	–	83	16	1	<1	–	73	96	335	55
Black	65*	33*	–	1	–	74	26	–	–	–	65	66*	148	66
Grey	70	23	6	2	–	82	18	<1	–	–	no data	53	163	nd
Brown	69	31	–	–	–	80	18	1	<1	–	80	87	237	98
Silver	73	27	–	–	–	87	10	1	<1	1	75	99	243	44
Gold	90	10	–	–	–	87	13	<1	–	–	85	100	258	97
Bronze	88	9	–	–	3	85	13	1	–	<1	87	94	149	54

*Figures for Black based on TR patients seen during pilot, all others based on pre-pilot TR sample.

5.3.2 Comparative figures for aids fitted to TR patients prior to DR also appear in table 5.3. Although in very broad terms the pattern is much the same as for DR patients, in quite a number of Centres the proportion of series 10 aids fitted is somewhat lower, most notably at Green (71% compared to 92%), Blue(NH) (83% compared to 95%), Grey (70% compared to 82%), and Silver (73% compared to 87%).

5.3.3 However, the data on TR patients fitted towards the end of the project period indicates that the proportions of series 10 aids in this set are in many cases much closer to the figures for DR patients. From the interviews with technicians, it was suggested that at times the aids fitted depend as much upon what is available as it does upon audiological considerations, and it may be that the varying proportions reflect this rather than any differences in management practices.

5.3.4 A total of four private aids were fitted amongst the sample of TR patients prior to DR, with three of these being at Bronze; and expressed as a rate, this is about double that amongst DR patients. However, it should be noted that most Centres included the cost of the extra aids they expected to fit as a result of DR in their bids to be included in the research, and only costed for NHS aids. This may have mitigated against the fitting of private aids to DR patients.

6 Waiting Times

6.1 Introduction

6.1.1 For both the TR and DR routes of provision, there are two principal 'milestones' after referral by a GP. The first of these is the first appointment at the hospital or clinic, either for an ENT examination (TR patients) or for examination by a technician (DR patients). The second major milestone is the appointment for the actual fitting of the hearing aid. A minority of patients have additional appointments to these (e.g. DR patients who are cross-referred, cases where the ear impressions have to be done on a different day to the testing), but for the purposes of analysing waiting times these additional appointments have been excluded.

6.1.2 Waiting times will therefore be studied in three aspects: the wait from GP referral to examination; the wait from examination to fitting; and the total wait from GP referral to fitting. The distributions of waiting times are quite heavily skewed, with a minority of patients experiencing unusually long waits. From the interviews with staff and patients it was clear that the principal cause of this was patients not attending appointments and then being seen at a later date. Often illness caused a delay, and it is known that in one case a patient went abroad for a year between first appointment and fitting!

6.1.3 Because of the skew in the distributions, it was felt that the computation of means would not be the most appropriate approach to this data, as the long tails would tend to inflate the means and misrepresent the experience of most patients. Therefore, the median, which is far less influenced by skew, was adopted as a more appropriate measure of 'average' waiting times.

6.1.4 With the exception of Black, all of the Centres took on extra clerical and/or technical support at the start of their DR service. This clearly had implications for waiting times, and these are discussed after the analysis of waiting times themselves has been presented. Also considered is the impact of the evaluation process itself.

6.2 Waiting times for TR patients

6.2.1 Waiting times from GP referral to ENT examination for the samples of TR patients appear in table 6.1. Prior to the project period there was a great deal of variation between Centres: four Centres – Orange, Green, Black, and Brown – had very short median waiting times, of 8 or 9 weeks; while at the other extreme, the median wait at Yellow was 40 weeks, at White it was 51

Table 6.1   Median waiting times from GP referral to first hospital appointment (in weeks)

| | TR prior to pilot | Second TR sample | Direct Referral | | | | Corresponding sample sizes | | | |
			1st third	Mid third	Last third	1st TR	2nd TR	First DR	Mid DR	Last DR
Orange	9 weeks	13 weeks	no data	no data	8 weeks	99	70	no data	no data	49
Red	70	22	36	18	9	89	77	10	47	41
Yellow	40	11	25	9	5	94	44	106	73	49
Green	8	9	4	3	6	95	71	52	67	66
Blue(NH)	20	33	3	4	4	88	65	88	88	83
Blue(PD)	not applicable		6	7	6	na	na	125	120	124
White	51	18	3	4	4	51	45	80	153	124
Black	6*	6	3	4	8	na	55	51	64	43
Grey	22	no data	5	8	3	49	nd	77	41	31
Brown	9	13	5	7	4	74	79	62	139	35
Silver	27	39	2	3	6	94	45	69	122	98
Gold	17	24	4	6	7	92	92	45	78	136
Bronze	17	19	5	5	6	69	54	27	47	60

*This figure for Black is what the Centre reported prior to the pilot.

weeks, and at Red 70 weeks. The average median wait for TR patients across all Centres was 37 weeks.

6.2.2 It was thought that the introduction of DR might shorten TR waiting times by removing patients from the ENT queue. However, the median waiting times for TR patients in the latter part of the project period do not really bear this out. While it is true that waiting times for an ENT appointment have dropped considerably in the three Centres which had the longest waits initially; Red, Yellow, and White; it is known that Red was operating a waiting list initiative scheme when the project started, specifically to reduce queues, and that Yellow transferred most of the patients queuing for ENT hearing aid clinics into the DR system. Apart from these three Centres TR waiting times for an ENT examination are actually higher – albeit in most cases only by a small amount – towards the end of the project at all other places bar Black (where they remained static).

6.2.3 Median waiting times from ENT examination to fitting of the aid appear in table 6.2. Six Centres show a reduction in this wait over the course of the project, while 5 show an increase. What may be happening here is that at some Centres the additional technical staff taken on at the start of the project provided enough capacity to reduce the waiting time for fitting for TR patients, as well as coping with the influx of DR patients. At other Centres, however, the additional staff have not proved sufficient, and waiting times for fitting have crept up.

6.2.4 A comparison of the wait from examination to fitting with that from GP to examination indicates that at most Centres the wait for fitting is the shorter of the two, often by a considerable amount. In the pre-pilot period, it was shorter at 9 Centres and longer at 3. The Centres where it was longer (Black, Grey, Brown) in fact all operated TR systems where large propor-

Table 6.2 Median waiting times from first appointment to fitting (in weeks)

	TR prior to pilot	Second TR sample	Direct Referral			Corresponding sample sizes				
			1st third	Mid third	Last third	1st TR	2nd TR	First DR	Mid DR	Last DR
Orange	5 weeks	8 weeks	no data	no data	6 weeks	98	70	no data	no data	49
Red	5	19	7	17	10	95	89	11	43	38
Yellow	3	2	2	2	2	93	40	104	70	44
Green	4	5	5	5	4	100	70	47	59	48
Blue(NH)	14	12	4	5	5	97	79	89	87	80
Blue(PD)	not applicable		5	6	3	na	na	121	110	112
White	13	5	3	4	4	95	58	77	145	113
Black	10*	15	10	10	7	na	65	43	61	35
Grey	36	no data	7	7	9	54	no data	70	52	33
Brown	25	4	5	5	4	81	92	59	130	39
Silver	6	5	2	3	6	98	45	58	190	76
Gold	5	3	4	4	3	98	93	44	80	133
Bronze	12	20	4	6	9	73	54	39	45	61

*This figure for Black is what the Centre reported prior to the pilot.

tions of patients had the hearing test and impressions on a different day to the ENT examination, and this is the principal reason why the wait for fitting is longer at these places. Excepting these, it is clear that the main factor in TR waiting times – particularly, very long waiting times – is the wait for an ENT examination.

6.2.5 Waiting times from GP referral to fitting (table 6.3) show the same mixed pattern as the previous tables. During the pilot period overall TR waits declined at four places, and increased at seven.

Table 6.3 Median waiting times from GP referral to fitting (in weeks)

	TR prior to pilot	Second TR sample	Direct Referral			Corresponding sample sizes				
			1st third	Mid third	Last third	1st TR	2nd TR	First DR	Mid DR	Last DR
Orange	15 weeks	21 weeks	no data	no data	13 weeks	98	70	no data	no data	49
Red	76	40	43	34	17	95	89	11	43	38
Yellow	42	14	28	13	7	93	40	104	70	44
Green	12	15	9	8	9	100	70	47	59	48
Blue(NH)	35	49	8	9	9	97	79	89	87	80
Blue(PD)	not applicable		10	13	9	na	na	121	110	112
White	65	24	7	8	8	95	58	77	145	113
Black	16*	22	14	14	15	na	65	43	61	35
Grey	62	no data	13	16	12	54	no data	70	52	33
Brown	35	18	10	12	10	81	92	59	130	39
Silver	37	43	5	7	12	98	45	58	190	76
Gold	23	28	8	10	10	98	93	44	80	133
Bronze	30	36	8	12	16	73	54	39	45	61

*This figure for Black is what the Centre reported prior to the pilot.

6.2.6 In table 6.4 figures are given for the proportions of TR patients who had very long waits – a year or more – between being referred by their GP and being fitted with the hearing aid. It can be seen that at some Centres the proportion waiting a year or more was very high initially, particularly at Red (92%), White (69%), Grey (76%) and Silver (42%). At the end of the project period, the number of patients waiting this long had dropped quite dramatically at Red (down to 13%), White (down to 2%), and Silver (7%). Unfortunately, Grey did not provide any data for this period. At only one Centre was there a substantial increase in TR patients waiting a long time, this was Blue(NH) where the proportion increased from 14% to 42%. Over all (comparable) Centres combined, the average proportion of TRs waiting a year or more declined from 24% to 9%, though how much of this reduction was due to the introduction of DR it is impossible to say.

Table 6.4
Percentages of TR patients waiting a year or more for the hearing aid

	Prior to pilot	Towards end of pilot	Sample size Prior	Towards end
Orange	3%	3%	98	69
Red	92	13	89	74
Yellow	4	–	92	44
Green	1	5	95	67
Blue(NH)	14	42	87	64
Blue(PD)	not applicable		not applicable	
White	69	2	92	44
Black	no data	2	no data	56
Grey	76	no data	49	no data
Brown	5	–	67	80
Silver	42	7	92	45
Gold	1	3	91	93
Bronze	12	11	74	54

6.3 Waiting times for DR patients, and comparison with TR waiting times

6.3.1 With regard to the waiting times for DR patients, it should be noted that at the start of the projects there was, of-course, no queue for this system. Consequently, it was to be expected that initially DR patients would experience very short waiting times. The important issue, therefore, is how quickly, and by how much, did the queue develop and waiting times increase. To address this question, the total time over which each project ran was divided into three equal time periods, and median waiting times derived separately for each.

6.3.2 The median waiting times from GP referral to first appointment appear in table 6.1. It will be observed that, contrary to the rest, Red and Yellow show very high waiting times for the initial period. Red selected patients for DR from the details given in GP letters, and it seems clear from the initial waiting time that they included many patients referred some considerable time before the start of the project. Yellow did the same thing by transferring patients who were in the queue for the ENT hearing aid clinic over to the DR scheme. In this respect, both Centres were operating against instructions they received prior to implementation of the schemes. In the event, however, the policies adopted produced worthwhile results in that the waiting times for both DR and TR patients at these Centres declined considerably over the course of the pilot period.

6.3.3 With regard to the other Centres, the variation in waiting times between one period and the next is generally quite small, and most of it is probably due to sampling variation. During the final period, the longest median wait anywhere for a first appointment was just 9 weeks, and at four Centres it was still only a month or less. In all but one Centre, DR patients at this time were still enjoying a shorter waiting time than comparable TR patients. The exception was Black, where the TR wait was 6 weeks, and the DR 8 weeks. Over all (comparable) Centres combined, the average median wait from GP to first appointment in the final period was 19 weeks for TR patients and 6 weeks for DR patients.

6.3.4 Median waits from first appointment to fitting are given in table 6.2. At nearly all Centres, DR patients experienced fairly short delays: there were just four Centres where, at any time, the wait was longer than 2 months. The wait experienced by DRs towards the end of the pilots was comparable to the TR wait at six Centres, while at four others it was shorter.

6.3.5 The median waiting times for the total process from GP referral to fitting for DR patients appear in table 6.3. Setting aside the 'special cases' of Red and Yellow, waiting times for the final period were very much the same as at the start in all but two Centres. These are Silver and Bronze, and in both cases waiting times have approximately doubled (from 5 weeks to 12 weeks at Silver, and 8 weeks to 16 weeks at Bronze). However, these waits are only fractionally on the high side compared to the other Centres.

6.3.6 The reason for the increase at Silver is not known. The Centre did not report that at any time it suffered from excessive workload or number of referrals (see section 12.3). However, the Centre did delay the fitting of some DR patients to make them available for interview by the evaluators (this is discussed more fully below), and it is possible that at least part of the longer wait for the last period is due to this. Bronze suffered financial problems during the last three months of the pilot, such that they were only able to do 'essential' fittings in this period, and this is the reason why their wait increased.

6.3.7 Compared to the waits for TR patients, the final period waits for DRs are shorter at all Centres. The average median wait for TRs (comparable Centres only) was 28 weeks, and for DRs it was 11 weeks.

6.4 Possible effects of the evaluation process on waiting times

6.4.1 There were two ways in which the evaluation process could have affected waiting times. Firstly, the evaluation generated a large amount of form-filling and other paperwork for technical staff. Secondly, some Centres 'held back' the fitting of some patients so that there would be sufficient available when the evaluators visited to interview.

6.4.2 However, both of these effects would have acted principally to increase the wait under DR. Also, neither affected the TR wait for an ENT examination, and in most cases this was the major part of the overall wait for TR patients. Therefore the basic conclusion that waiting times were shorter under DR is not affected.

6.5 Staff changes at the start of the projects and implications for waiting times

6.5.1 All of the Centres received funds to implement their DR schemes. All but one (Black) used at least part of this money to purchase additional hours of clerical and/or technical staff support for the Hearing Aid Centre. The hours purchased (in some cases new staff, in others more hours for existing staff) are listed in table 6.5.

Table 6.5

Hours per week of staff support purchased from pilot project funding

	Clerical staff	Technical staff
Orange	18 hours per week	37.5 MTO3
Red	37.5	–
Yellow	20	37.5 Student + 8 hours private dispenser
Green	37.5	19 MTO3
Blue	6	20 MTO3 + 10 Patients per week seen by private dispenser
White	22	75 MTO3
Black	–	–
Grey	unknown	unknown mixture of private dispenser and NHS tech time
Brown	–	22.5 MTO2 + 6 hours private dispenser
Silver	12	8 MTO3
Gold	37.5	37.5 Student
Bronze	–	20 MTO3

6.5.2 The extra staff hours were specifically to deal with the expected extra work under DR. Judging from the waiting times, the majority of Centres coped with this well. There were only two (Silver and Bronze) where DR waiting times notably increased over the pilot period, but the former did not rate the workload as a problem, and at the latter the problem had been with funding to purchase hearing aids.

6.5.3 With regard to TR patients, the extra staff hours also had some influence here. Excluding Red (which as had been said, ran a waiting list initiative scheme), there were three Centres where the overall TR waiting time (GP to fitting) dropped substantially over the project: Yellow, White, and Brown. Yellow transferred long-waiting TR patients to the DR scheme, and the extra staff hours must have helped here; part of the reduction at White was due to a reduction in time between ENT exam and fitting, which is dictated by availability of technicians; and all of the reduction at Brown was due to the same factor.

6.5.4 It seems likely that without the extra staff hours many Centres would not have been able to maintain the short waiting times for DR patients, or (where it occurred) reduce TR waits. After the end of the pilot period, some Centres lost staff hours as a result of Department of Health funding for the projects coming to an end (in other cases the health authority took over the funding). What happened to waiting times after this point is unfortunately not known.

6.6 Summary and discussion

6.6.1 At all Centres directly referred patients experienced shorter waiting times than those coming through the traditional system of provision. In the latter part of the pilot period the average wait from GP to fitting for a DR patient was 11 weeks, and for a TR patient it was 28 weeks. Although at most Centres the average wait experienced by TRs actually increased a little over the period, those Centres with very long TR waits reduced these substantially, such that the overall proportion of TRs having very long waits (a year or more) declined considerably, from 24% to 9%.

6.6.2 Results from the survey of pre-existing DR schemes were very similar to these (see Part II, section 32). In this survey the average wait under DR was 13 weeks, and under TR it was 26 weeks (based on 16 Centres operating both systems).

6.6.3 However, there were two pre-existing schemes where the wait under DR had grown to be longer than under TR, and in both cases this was due to reductions in the number of technicians. At another 5 Centres DR had either been suspended for a time or stopped completely because of a shortage of technical staff. Also, since the end of the pilot period one of the pilot Centres – Bronze – has been forced to suspend its scheme for the same reason.

6.6.4 It is clear from this that while Direct Referral can reduce waiting times substantially, the continuance of this very much depends upon staffing levels at the Hearing Aid Centre being maintained.

7 Technician Examinations of DR Patients

7.1 Details of the data collected

7.1.1 Technicians (including the private dispensers) completed a pro-forma on each directly referred patient that they examined (appendix I.I.II). This recorded the findings of the history-taking and ear-examination, and the action(s) undertaken.

7.1.2 The form incorporated a check-list of examination items, based upon the guidelines for assessing Direct Referral patients produced by the Liaison Group for Technicians, Therapists and Scientists in Audiology (TTSA, these guidelines appear in appendix I.III). However, the pro-forma was not intended to act as a schedule for directing the examination, but purely as a recording instrument. How each Centre structured the examination procedure was up to them to decide.

7.1.3 Each of the items on the checklist (e.g. earache, tinnitus, active discharge) could be ticked as being either 'Significant' or 'Present'. 'Significant' implied that the item was serious enough for the patient to be cross-referred to ENT; 'Present' meant that the item was apparent, but did not require ENT inspection. There was also a space on the form for the technician to write down any significant factors not covered by the checklist.

7.1.4 The presence of wax was not included as a checklist item. This was because wax management was given a separate section of its own on a companion form. However, given the number of times that wax was written in as a factor in cross-referral, with hindsight it would have been advantageous to include it in the checklist.

7.1.5 The list of possible actions which could be undertaken was as follows: (a) Degree of loss does not warrant hearing aid; (b) Appropriate to fit hearing aid; (c) Cross-refer to ENT; (d) Review patient's ears again at later date; and (e) 'Other'. More than one action could be indicated.

7.2 Grades of technicians examining DR patients
(table 7.1)

7.2.1 Senior NHS technicians (i.e. MTO3 and above) accounted for the great majority of examinations, some 73% of the total. The largest contribution was by MTO3s, who did 50% of all examinations. There were just two Centres where technicians below this grade were involved: at Grey, technicians of grade MTO2 accounted for just 11% of the examinations, while at Brown 81% were conducted by staff of this grade. At both of these Centres,

Table 7.1 Grades of technicians who examined DR patients (figures in percentages)

	Trainee	MTO2	MTO3	MTO4	MTO5	Aud. Scientist	Private Dispenser	Sample size
Orange				not known			–	
Red	–	–	42%	49%	9%	–	–	105
Yellow	–	–	42	–	39	–	19	241
Green	–	–	98	–	2	–	–	188
Blue(NH)	–	–	84	14	2	–	–	276
Blue(PD)	–	–	–	–	–	–	100	371
White	–	–	82	18	–	–	–	376
Black	–	–	50	50	–	–	–	171
Grey	–	11	32	3	–	–	53	175
Brown	1	81	1	–	–	1	15	283
Silver	–	–	91	–	9	–	–	299
Gold	–	–	38	37	26	–	–	266
Bronze	–	–	36	50	14	–	–	168
Overall	<1%	9%	50%	15%	8%	<1%	19%	2919

the MTO2s involved were at the top of the scale, and had many years experience of seeing hearing aid patients. Also at Brown, 4 patients were examined by a trainee technician. However, it was noted that this was under supervision from one of the senior staff.

7.2.2 Private dispensers were involved at four Centres. They conducted 15% of examinations at Brown, 19% at Yellow, 53% at Grey, and 100% at Blue(PD). Overall, private dispensers did 19% of all examinations.

7.3 Rates of various actions decided on by technicians

7.3.1 The various forms of action decided upon by technicians who examined DR patients are summarized in table 7.2. Red used their own pro-formas, which did not record the actions undertaken (apart from whether an aid was to be fitted). For each Centre, the percentages summed across all actions add to more than 100%, because in some cases more than one action was indicated. Patients who were found to already have a hearing aid when they attended have been excluded from the analysis.

7.3.2 *Loss too low*. These were cases where the technician decided that the patient's hearing was good enough to make fitting an aid unnecessary. At most Centres this was a very small proportion, though at Silver and Brown it was somewhat higher, particularly at the latter where one in every ten patients fell into this category.

7.3.3 *Patient did not want aid*. There were a small number of cases, typically 1% or 2% at each Centre, where although the technician felt that an aid would be appropriate, the patient themselves decided that they did not want one, at least for the time being. In addition (and not included in these rates) a

Table 7.2 Actions resulting from technician examinations of DR patients (figures in percentages)

	Loss too low to warrant aid	Patient did not want aid	Appropriate to fit aid	Cross-refer to ENT	Review ears at later date	Dewax needed	Refer back to GP	Sample size
Orange	6%	2%	84%	11%	4%	unknown	–	101
Red				information incomplete				
Yellow	6	2	92	39	2	21	–	243
Green	2	<1	76	28	<1	8	–	190
Blue(NH)	1	–	98	15	4	2	–	276
Blue(PD)	3	<1	95	3	<1	–	–	371
White	2	<1	85	24	2	3	–	377
Black	4	2	88	19	<1	11	–	171
Grey	–	–	99	13	1	10	–	177
Brown	10	1	88	5	1	4	<1	284
Silver	8	<1	84	9	1	9	2	304
Gold	2	<1	87	44	3	15	<1	266
Bronze	6	1	87	7	–	10	–	172

few others changed their minds and refused the aid later in the provision process.

7.3.4 *Appropriate to fit aid*. At every Centre, the technicians decided to fit hearing aids to the great majority of patients. This ranged from 76% at Green, up to 99% at Grey. The exceptions were cases where either the hearing loss was very low, the patient did not want an aid, or the patient was cross-referred to ENT prior to a decision being made. With regard to the latter, the great majority of these cases were, at the end of the day, sent back to the Hearing Aid Centre for fitting.

7.3.5 Policy with respect to the fitting of cross-referrals varied somewhat. Technicians in some Centres were more cautious about fitting cross-referrals than in others. This was particularly true at Green, where the decision was left to the ENT doctor seeing the cross-referral in the great majority of cases. This policy may have been the result of an experience early in the project, when an ENT doctor complained about an aid being fitted to a patient with otitis media prior to him seeing them. An additional consideration is that once they have obtained the aid, a number of cross-referred patients refuse to return for the ENT examination – this point is considered more fully in a later section.

7.3.6 *Cross-referral to ENT*. Rates of cross-referral varied considerably between Centres. The lowest rate was just 3% of patients at Blue(PD), and the highest was 44%, at Gold. Rates for the other Centres are scattered right across this range, and there is no figure which might be called 'typical'. There are several reasons why the differences are so large. Firstly, there are definite differences between areas in the actual incidence of ear pathology: this became very clear when the external specialists made their visits, as both of them commented on the wide variation in rates of disease they discovered in different Centres.

7.3.7 Secondly, there are differences in the GPs referring to each project. It is not possible to say whether GPs in some areas did a better job of selecting patients for DR than in others – though this could be true – but it is true that some Centres went to greater lengths to make sure GPs understood the criteria and followed them.

7.3.8 Thirdly, cross-referral rates tend to be higher in those Centres where ENT consultants showed an active and definite interest in the project, and co-operated fully in its operation. In those Centres where ENT showed less interest, and co-operation was more difficult to obtain, it seems that technicians either adopted more relaxed standards, or were more reluctant to make cross-referrals. It must be emphasised that this is a *general* observation, and is not true in every case.

7.3.9 It is of interest to compare the cross-referral rates for NHS technicians with those for private dispensers. In three of the four Centres where private dispensers were involved, their rate was lower than that of NHS technicians at the same Centre. The difference is particularly dramatic at Yellow, where the dispenser rate was 4% compared to 47% for NHS technicians; and it was also high at Blue; 3% compared to 15%. In both cases the difference is significant at the 1% level (chi-squared test). At Brown, the rate was 2% as against to 6%, but this is not significantly different. At Grey the dispenser and the NHS technicians had the same rate, 13%.

7.3.10 *Review.* The numbers of patients that technicians wanted to review at a later date were low in all Centres (note that 'review' does not include the standard follow-ups received by most hearing-aid patients). The most common reason for wanting to review a patient was where the hearing loss was borderline, and might be expected to deteriorate – making an aid appropriate -in the not too distant future. Another common reason was where the audiometry was doubtful (e.g. the patient had a cold), and needed to be repeated.

7.3.11 *Dewax needed.* The rates reported in this column include all patients whom technicians decided were in need of wax removal; whether they were dewaxed that day, sent back to their GP for dewax, or given a later appointment for dewaxing. There were a number of other cases where technicians recorded that wax was present, but did not indicate that they had advised a dewax. These are not included in the rates. The highest rate was at Yellow, where 21% of patients needed wax removal, this is followed by Gold, with 15%. The lowest was at Blue(PD), where no patients at all were referred for dewaxing. The rate for the NHS scheme at Blue was also very low, just 2%. However, 76% of patients at this Centre reported being dewaxed by their GP prior to attending, more than at any other Centre (see table 16.1).

7.3.12 There were many cases where technicians recommended hearing aids and took ear impressions prior to a patient being dewaxed. Also, it is clear that several patients managed in this way and told to return to their GP for dewax did not do so, as the wax was still present when they returned for their ENT safety check. In two instances, one at Green and one at Blue, ENT doctors expressed concern on the pro-forma that impressions had been taken and aids fitted to ears blocked with wax.

7.3.13 In addition to this, there were a number of cases where technicians stated on the pro-forma that they could not see one or both ear-drums due to wax, but fitted the patient and did not cross-refer them. Of a total across all Centres of 50 instances where a drum could not be seen, 23 were cross-referred, and 27 not cross-referred. However, there were big differences between Centres: at one Centre there were 14 cases, and all were cross-referred; whereas at another only 4 out of a total of 22 were crossed. It must also be borne in mind that the pro-forma did not specifically ask technicians to record whether they could see the drum, and these instances are only known of because a 'voluntary' comment was made on the form. It is quite possible therefore, that the actual number of such cases was higher than this.

7.3.14 *Sent back to GP (not for dewax)*. The final column in table 7.2 refers to a small number of patients whom technicians felt needed to go back to their GP. Only three Centres reported any such instances, and at two of these (Brown and Gold) there was just one such case, whereas at Silver there was 6. In all of these cases the patients had ear conditions other than simple hearing loss which should have excluded them from being directly referred. At Brown and Gold the cases were one of dizziness and one of ear infection, which the technicians apparently felt should be managed by the GP rather than ENT. At Silver the cases were two patients with vertigo, two with Menière's disease, and two with multiple ear conditions. The vertigo cases were fitted with aids anyway, and in some other cases the GP was advised to re-refer the patient to ENT.

7.3.15 No Centre reported any instance of a technician referring a patient back to their GP for a medical condition unrelated to the ear. However, the pro-forma did not explicitly ask about such cases, and so it is possible that they did occur but were not recorded.

7.4 Reasons for cross-referring

7.4.1 Technicians gave a wide variety of reasons for cross-referring patients. These are listed in table 7.3 along with the proportion of cases (across all Centres combined) in which they occurred. In any one instance of cross-referral, more than one reason may have been specified. Far and away the most common reasons were asymmetric loss (present in 36% of cross-referrals), and conductive loss (33%). Apart from these, only three other factors were significant in more than 10% of cross-referrals: Tinnitus (14%); vertigo (12%), and loss in one ear only (11%). Other reasons of note were perforations (9%), and a history of discharge (9%).

7.4.2 Quite a number of reasons were given which were not covered by the checklist of TTSA guideline items. The most common of these was where the view of the eardrum was obscured (4% of cases). In most cases this was due to wax, but there were a few where the canals were very narrow, or a heavy growth of hair in the ear blocked the view. Wax, in most cases associ-

Table 7.3

Technicians – reasons given for cross-referring

Total number of cross-referrals = 530

	Number of cases crossed for this	As a % of all cross-referrals
Checklist items (Based on TTSA guidelines)		
HISTORY ITEMS		
Sudden onset of loss	22	4.2%
Fluctuating loss	14	2.6
Loss in one ear only	57	10.8
Vertigo	66	12.4
Tinnitus	74	14.0
Earache	35	6.6
History of discharge	45	8.5
EXAMINATION ITEMS		
Active discharge	30	5.7
Diseased canal	19	3.6
Perforated drum	47	8.9
Inflamed drum	17	3.2
Scarred drum	36	6.8
AUDIOMETRY ITEMS		
Asymmetric loss	192	36.2
Conductive loss	175	33.0
Reasons not covered by checklist		
View of drum obscured	23	4.3
Wax	21	4.0
Abnormal drum	23	4.3
Retracted drum	18	3.4
Typanometric abnormality	17	3.2
Audiometric abnormality	17	3.2
Pressure/blockage/pain/irritation	9	1.7
Polyps/growth in ear canal	7	1.3
Noise exposure	7	1.3
Mastoid cavity	4	0.8
Abnormal pinna	3	0.6
Attic retraction pocket	2	0.4
Fluid	2	0.4
Balance problems	7	1.3
Non-auditory problems	7	1.3

Note: In any one case more than one reason may be given, therefore percentages add to more than 100%.

ated with an obscured view, was also given as a reason in 4% of cases. Other relatively frequently cited non-guideline factors were: an abnormal looking drum (4%); a retracted drum (3%); typanometric abnormalities (3%); and audiometric abnormalities (3%).

8 ENT Safety-Check Examinations of DR Patients

8.1 Arrangements for safety-checks

8.1.1 One of the conditions for involvement as a pilot Centre was that all DR patients seen under the pilot scheme should receive a safety-check by an ENT doctor. The only exceptions to this were domiciliary patients too infirm to attend the hospital.

8.1.2 The local ENT doctors who conducted safety-checks completed a pro-forma for each patient they examined (appendix I.I.III). This was similar to the pro-formas that technicians used, incorporating the same check-list of items based on the TTSA guidelines, but with a slightly different list of possible actions which could be undertaken. Specifically, this list was: (a) loss too low to warrant aid; (b) appropriate to fit aid; (c) further investigation required; (d) medical intervention required; (e) review patients' ears again at later date; and (f) other. The form also included a section concerned with the potential seriousness of any medical conditions identified. However, this section was inconsistently completed, and so has not been analyzed.

8.2 Patients who did not receive a safety-check

8.2.1 At every Centre there was a proportion of DR patients who did not receive an ENT safety-check. It was agreed early on, as part of the methodology, that infirm patients seen as domiciliary visits could be excluded from having a safety-check. Also, a few patients died before the safety examination. In addition, most patients who were found to already have a hearing aid were not given a safety-check, and it appears that some Centres did not arrange safety-checks for many patients where the technician decided that the hearing was adequate (presumably, they did not feel justified in asking the patient to return for this alone). Even excluding the above categories, however, there were a number of other patients who were either too ill, or refused to attend the ENT check.

8.2.2 Of particular concern are those patients whom technicians cross-referred, but who did not return for the ENT examination. The worst case appears to have been at Blue(PD), where 5 out of a total of 11 cross-referrals did not attend ENT. This is exceptional however, as rates for the other Centres were much lower than this: e.g. Blue(NH) 12%; White 7%; Black 3%. Most, if not all, of these patients were fitted with the aid prior to the ENT appointment, and it seems that once they had obtained the hearing aid a proportion were unwilling to return again. This is worrying because these are the patients who most need an ENT examination.

8.3 Grades of ENT doctors doing safety checks

(table 8.1)

8.3.1 The grades of ENT doctors who conducted the safety-checks varied considerably from one Centre to another. In nearly all Centres a good variety of doctors was involved, ranging from consultants down to SHOs, and even house officers in a few cases. There was just one project, Black, at which virtually all of the safety- checks were made by a single doctor (a consultant).

Table 8.1 Grades of ENT doctors who conducted safety-checks (figures in percentages)

	House Officer	Senior house Officer	Clinical Assistant	Registrar	Senior Clin. Assistant	Senior Registrar	Consultant	Sample size
Orange				not known				
Red	–	2%	20%	29%	–	14%	35%	102
Yellow	–	>99	–	–	–	–	<1	234
Green	15	19	–	12	–	26	29	184
Blue(NH)	–	–	>99	–	–	–	<1	235
Blue(PD)	–	–	>99	–	–	–	<1	226
White	9	31	–	11	–	7	44	335
Black	–	<1	–	<1	1	<1	97	146
Grey	–	–	–	3	–	<1	96	171
Brown	<1	35	–	37	–	7	21	249
Silver	–	84	–	–	–	–	16	155
Gold	–	–	–	78	–	4	18	266
Bronze	–	8	–	13	–	74	6	134
Overall	2%	25%	20%	17%	<1%	9%	28%	2437

8.3.2 Taking 'senior' ENT doctor to mean a consultant, senior registrar, or senior clinical assistant, at five Centres the majority of checks were done by senior doctors: Green (55%); White (51%); Black (97%); Grey (97%) and Bronze (80%). Red is just out of this group, with 49%. Towards the opposite end of the scale, at two Centres SHOs conducted almost all the checks; Yellow (99%), and Silver (84%). The lowest grade, house officers, were involved to a small degree at three Centres: Green (15%); White (9%); and Brown (less than 1%).

8.3.3 Over all Centres combined, consultants accounted for the single largest percentage of patients, 28%. SHOs were next, at 25%, followed by clinical assistants at 20%. House officers accounted for around 2%.

8.4 Rates of various actions decided on by ENT doctor

(table 8.2)

8.4.1 *Loss too low to warrant aid.* The numbers of DR patients considered by doctors not to require a hearing aid were low everywhere, the highest figure being 9%, at Yellow. However, the figures in most cases are somewhat underestimated, as a disproportionate number of patients passed by technicians as having adequate hearing were not seen by ENT: just 54% of such patients received a safety-check. This proportion varied considerably from Centre to Centre, and so for some places (most notably Blue, White, Silver, Bronze) the figure is quite a bit lower than it otherwise would have been.

Table: 8.2 Actions resulting from ENT safety-checks on DR patients (figures in percentages)

	Loss too low to warrant aid	Appropriate to fit aid	Investigate /treat	Review again at later date	Dewax needed	Action on non-ear problem	Other	Sample size
Orange			— no data —					
Red	2%	96%	1%	1%	0%	0%	0%	106
Yellow	9	90	2	7	<1	<1	0	237
Green	4	88	11	5	4	0	1	186
Blue(NH)	0	>99	2	<1	5	<1	0	236
Blue(PD)	<1	98	1	<1	5	0	<1	229
White	2	95	3	2	<1	0	<1	337
Black	5	92	5	2	2	<1	0	148
Grey	0	99	5	2	5	0	1	173
Brown	8	91	10	4	<1	<1	1	251
Silver	2	94	3	4	<1	0	0	162
Gold	2	97	9	6	6	0	0	266
Bronze	<1	>99	<1	0	<1	0	0	134

8.4.2 *Appropriate to fit hearing aid.* The proportions of patients for whom ENT doctors recommended hearing aids was very high at all Centres, the lowest being 88%, at Green, while at three other Centres it was over 99%. For the reason given above, however, the figures for some Centres are a few percentage points higher than they would otherwise have been.

8.4.3 *Further investigation/medical treatment needed.* These two categories have been combined because at most Centres the numbers were small. In nine out of twelve projects, the percentage of patients requiring further investigation or treatment was 5% or less. The three exceptions were Green (11%), Brown (10%), and Gold (9%).

8.4.4 *Review patient again at a later date.* There were a broad variety of reasons for a doctor wishing to do a review. The most important, and most common, was where there was a suggestion of pathology, and the doctor wanted to check on any future development of this. Other reasons included checking on a currently quiescent condition, or on a discharging ear, mastoid, or perforation; looking for further deterioration in hearing; or making a future appointment to give specific advice on tinnitus or another ENT problem. Rates of patients requiring review vary from 0% up to 7%.

8.4.5 *Dewax needed.* The 'Dewax' category includes all cases where the ENT doctor either carried out a dewax, or noted that a dewax was needed. The figures here combine cases where the technician had failed to arrange wax removal previously, and also cases where the removal was done at the safety appointment on the behest of the technician. Patients who were dewaxed prior to the safety-check are not included. Figures are low at all Centres, the highest being 6%, at Gold, while at six Centres it was less than 1%.

8.4.6 *Action needed on a non-ear problem.* There were just four instances of a condition being identified as needing intervention that was not to do with the ear. They were each at a different Centre, and were: a voice problem at Blue; nasal problem at Black; thyroid swelling at Brown; and throat problem at Yellow.

8.4.7 *Other actions.* The category of 'Other' covers just a handful of patients where any of the following was recorded: referral to another hospital department or speciality; patient needed ENT advice; ENT doctor critical of patients management by technician. These types of action were not included in the pro-forma checklist, but were written in the space for 'other' actions. It may be therefore, that the figures underestimate the actual incidence of such cases.

8.5 All types of ENT action combined

8.5.1 Table 8.3 presents figures for all types of ENT action combined. The first column covers all cases where ENT wanted no further management of the patient, other than possibly a dewax. The second column pertains to all cases needing further management, whether investigation, treatment, review, referral on, ENT advice, or where the ENT doctor was critical of the technicians management of the case. The resulting figures therefore represent fairly severe estimates of the proportions requiring further management.

Table 8.3
Percentages of patients requiring further ENT management

	No further management /dewax only	Further management required	Sample size
Orange	——— no data ———		
Red	98%	2	106
Yellow	91	9	237
Green	85	15	186
Blue(NH)	97	3	236
Blue(PD)	98	2	229
White	96	4	337
Black	95	5	148
Grey	93	7	173
Brown	86	14	251
Silver	94	6	162
Gold	88	12	266
Bronze	——— not known* ———		134

*ENT doctors at Bronze did not complete pro-formas for cross-referred patients.

8.5.2 The proportions of patients for whom further management was required varied from 2% at Red and Blue(PD), up to 15% at Green. (ENT doctors at Bronze did not complete pro-formas for cross-referred patients, and so the figure for this Centre is unknown.) Two other Centres had notably high proportions: Brown at 14% and Gold at 12%.

8.6 Reasons for ENT doctors wanting further patient management
(table 8.4)

8.6.1 The reasons given by ENT doctors for wanting further management of a patient have been divided into those covered by the TTSA guidelines, and those outside of the guidelines. With respect to guideline items, the most common by far were asymmetric loss (47% of cases) and conductive loss (25%). These were also the most common reasons for cross-referral cited by technicians (see 7.4.1). Of the other TTSA checklist items, those of most note are: loss in one ear only (19%); tinnitus (9%); scarred drum (8%); vertigo (7%); perforated drum (6%); and history of discharge (6%). With the exception of scarring, these factors were also the ones most frequently cited by technicians.

8.6.2 The list of factors which were not on the checklist is composed mainly of more specific diagnoses. Of particular interest are those which represent the more serious forms of middle ear disease: Otitis Media (6 cases); Chronic Suppurative Otitis Media (3 cases); Middle Ear Effusion (2 cases); Mastoiditis (1 case); Cholesteatoma (4 cases); Glue ear (1 case); Attic retraction pocket (4 cases); Attic disease (2 cases); and quiescent middle ear disease (7 cases). Altogether, these comprise a total of 27 different patients, which is 16% of all those requiring further management, or 1.1% of all patients examined.

Table 8.4

ENT doctors – reasons for further management

Total number requiring further management = 171

	Number of cases requiring further management for this	As a % of all requiring further management
Checklist items (Based on TTSA guidelines)		
HISTORY ITEMS		
Sudden onset of loss	7	4.1%
Fluctuating loss	3	1.8
Loss in one ear only	32	18.7
Vertigo	12	7.0
Tinnitus	16	9.4
Earache	2	1.2
History of discharge	10	5.8
EXAMINATION ITEMS		
Active discharge	6	3.5
Diseased canal	9	5.3
Perforated drum	11	6.4
Inflamed drum	2	1.2
Scarred drum	13	7.6
AUDIOMETRY ITEMS		
Asymmetric loss	80	46.8
Conductive loss	42	24.6
Items not on checklist		
Wax	3	1.8
Abnormal drum	3	1.8
Retracted drum	1	0.6
Typanometric abnormality	1	0.6
Audiometric abnormality	3	1.8
Noise exposure	3	1.8
Eczema	2	1.2
Otitis Externa	8	4.8
Debris	2	1.2
Wart in ear canal	1	0.6
Otitis Media	6	3.5
CSOM	3	1.8
Middle ear effusion	2	1.2
Mastoiditis	1	0.6
Cholesteatoma	4	2.3
Glue ear	1	0.6
Attic retraction pocket	4	2.3
Attic disease	2	1.2
Quiescent middle ear disease	7	4.1
Otosclerosis	4	2.3
Cochlear Otosclerosis	1	0.6
Ossicular discontinuity	1	0.6
Non-auditory problems	8	4.8
Patient needed ENT advice	3	1.8
Referred on	2	1.2
ENT critical of tech management	3	1.8

Note: More than one reason may be given, so percentages add to more than 100%

9 Patient Safety: Comparison of Technician and ENT Examinations

9.1 Introduction

9.1.1 The technician examinations of DR patients can be compared with the ENT safety-checks on the same patients in order to assess the safety of the DR procedure. Patients who were felt by ENT to require further management but who were not cross-referred by a technician, can be regarded as technician management failures: under a 'normal' DR system (i.e. without the ENT safety-check), these patients would not be seen by an ENT doctor at all, and might possibly miss out on important ENT management.

9.1.2 Comparing the outcomes of the two examinations provides a measure of the performance of technicians *relative to the decisions made by their own local doctors*. It is quite possible, however, that the doctors themselves make errors of management in some cases. An assessment of the safety of Direct Referral would not be complete unless this factor were also taken into account. The research project attempted to do this by having samples of DR and TR patients medically assessed by ENT specialists of high standing who were independent of any of the pilot Centres. The results from this exercise are presented and discussed in the chapter following this one.

9.2 Previous evaluations of the safety of Direct Referral

9.2.1 Four previously published studies have sought to address the issue of the safety of Direct Referral. In addition, two other studies have been reported in the form of letters in medical journals. All but one of the above, however, looked only at the referral performance of GPs, and did not examine an actual Direct Referral system.

9.2.2 The studies by Harries et al (1989), Watson and Crowther (1989), Bellini et al (1989), Campbell et al (1989), and Prinsley et al (1989); all investigated samples of patients who had been referred by GPs to ENT departments either for a hearing aid, or for assessment and treatment of hearing impairment. Four of these studies found quite significant amounts of ear pathology missed by GPs, and concluded that patients should continue to be assessed by ENT medical staff. The remaining study (Prinsley et al) while also finding that a sizable proportion of patients required further investigation or treatment, found none of these cases serious, and gave its support to a change in referral practice.

9.2.3 It is relevant to note that all of the studies mentioned above restricted themselves to consideration of otological conditions only. A number of investigators, however, have presented evidence that hearing loss in the elderly can be associated with non-otological medical conditions, most notably vascular and metabolic disorders and drug-induced ototoxicity (Griffin (1988), Johnsson and Hawkins (1972), Makishima (1978) and Lim and Stephens (1991)). For example, Lim and Stephens (1991) in a study of 80 elderly patients presenting with a hearing problem found that 46% had previously undiagnosed but treatable vascular or metabolic disorders, and that 30% were taking potentially ototoxic drugs. They note that if these conditions were treated hearing may perhaps be slightly improved and the likelihood of further deterioration reduced. These findings have implications for Direct Referral, because the conditions involved are not ones that audiological technicians could in any way be expected to detect.

9.2.4 All of the aforementioned studies of pathology in hearing aid patients are essentially audits of GP performance within the Traditional Referral framework. As such, all suffer the same major drawback: referring GPs are not particularly concerned about diagnosing the specific cause of a hearing loss, because they know that the patient is going to be examined at the hospital by an otolaryngologist. Under an actual DR system, where GPs are informed that they are expected to appropriately select patients and that these patients will not necessarily be seen by an ENT surgeon, they may act differently.

9.2.5 A study by Hawthorne et al (1991) is the only one to examine the performance of a DR system in operation. In this study, GPs were issued with a standard referral letter, incorporating a checklist of referral criteria. Out of the first 300 referrals, 225 were examined by both an audiology technician and an ENT surgeon, who assessed the same factors as the GP. The ENT surgeon considered 98 patients as suitable for Direct Referral, indicating that the GPs had failed to follow the criteria in 127 (56%) of cases. However, at the end of the day, 91% of the 225 patients received a hearing aid with no other management apart from wax removal. This led Hawthorne et al to conclude that GPs were referring accurately, even though they frequently failed to correctly assess the criteria (Hawthorne et al, 1991 p.826).

9.2.6 With regard to the performance of the technicians, all cases needing management other than just a hearing aid were correctly identified. The authors conclude from this that a Direct Referral system can be safe. However, they emphasis that reliance must be placed on the technical staffs' ability to detect ear disease, and not solely on the GP. In addition, they note that the technicians involved were senior staff with high levels of training and at least five years experience.

9.3 Time-lag between technician exam and safety-check

9.3.1 For practical reasons alone, it was inevitable that under the pilot projects some patients, at least, were going to experience a delay between being examined by the technician and then receiving their ENT check. It was clear from the beginning that this could cause some problems for the research, in that some patients might develop pathology during this period, resulting in a false discrepancy between what the technician found and the ENT conclusions.

9.3.2 In order to minimise the danger of this, Centres were asked to try to keep the time delay as short as possible. At six Centres the median delay was a month or less: Red, Yellow, Green, White, Grey, and Gold. Indeed, at Red, Yellow and Gold, the majority of patients had their safety-check the same day as their technician exam (88%, 63% and 78%, respectively). Contrasted to these, were four Centres where the median delay was 3 months or more: Blue(PD), Black, Brown, and Silver. Silver had the longest median delay of all, 15 weeks.

9.3.3 It is hard to say how much effect the delays could have had on the results. In two cases staff noted on the pro-formas that a pathology picked up by ENT was not present when the technician saw the patient. In one of these, for example, a 30db asymmetric loss developed between examinations. In order to take account of the delay – as far as is possible – it will be seen later in this chapter that all instances of serious discrepancy have been evaluated as to whether they could have been due to pathology developing between examinations.

9.4 Comparison of technician and ENT examinations

9.4.1 The outcomes of the ENT examinations have been categorised in relationship to the actions decided upon by technicians. Results are presented separately for those patients who were cross-referred and those who were not. The cases have been divided into four different categories. The first category 'No Further Management' covers those cases where the ENT doctor agreed completely with the technician in terms of the fitting (or otherwise) of an aid, and whether a dewax was required.

9.4.2 The second category 'Differed on aid only' includes all cases where the only difference concerned a detail about the fitting. These were cases where ENT felt an aid was not necessary, whereas the technician had fitted one, or vice versa; or where ENT said the aid would be better in the other ear, or that two aids should be fitted instead of one. These disagreements were generally minor, and several of them were actually the result of the patient having had experience of the aid. No instances were recorded of the ENT doctor saying that a different model or type of aid should be fitted.

9.4.3 The third category concerns those cases where the technician did not arrange wax removal, but the ENT doctor conducted a dewax or noted that one was needed.

9.4.4 The last category covers all those cases where ENT considered that the patient needed further management. This includes a broad variety of actions: further investigation; medical treatment; a review at a later date; referral to another speciality; ENT advice; and cases where the doctor was critical of the technicians management of the patient.

9.4.5 Unfortunately, two Centres had to be excluded from the present analysis: Orange, because none of the ENT examination forms were completed at that Centre; and Red, which failed to indicate which patients were cross-referred and which not.

9.5 ENT actions on cross-referred patients (table 9.1)

9.5.1 Looking firstly at patients who were cross-referred, the column in table 9.1 headed 'No Further Management' provides the percentages of cross-referred patients who presented nothing that ENT wanted to take action on. The percentages are nearly all high, with only Brown (40%) and Silver (50%) being less than 60%. This may suggest that a good proportion of DR patients were cross-referred unnecessarily. However, what is not known is how many of these patients had symptoms which, even though not significant, did need an ENT opinion.

Table 9.1
ENT actions on patients cross-referred by technicians

	Total crossed	No further management	Differ on aid only	Dewax only	Further management
Orange		———————— not known ————————			
Red		———————— not known ————————			
Yellow	90	80%	3%	0%	17%
Green	54	61	0	0	39
Blue(NH)	37	87	0	3	11
Blue(PD)	6	67	0	0	33
White	85	84	0	1	15
Black	32	78	0	0	22
Grey	22	68	0	0	32
Brown	15	40	0	0	60
Silver	14	50	7	0	43
Gold	116	71	0	<1	28
Bronze	12	———————— no data* ————————			

*At Bronze, ENT doctors did not complete pro-formas for crossed patients

9.5.2 There were very few cases indeed where the ENT doctor differed with respect to the aid fitting, or where a dewax was required.

9.5.3 The percentages of cross-referred patients who needed further management ranged from 11% at Blue(NH), up to 60% at Brown, though this latter figure is based on a total of only 15 patients cross-referred. Other Centres with notably high percentages were Silver (43%) and Green (39%).

9.6 ENT actions on patients who were not cross-referred (table 9.2)

9.6.1 The figures for patients who were *not* cross-referred are perhaps more interesting. In a typical Direct Referral system, none of these patients would be seen by an ENT doctor, and any failures by the technicians would go unnoticed. The safety-checks in the pilot projects, however, allow us to gauge how many such failures there are likely to be.

9.6.2 With regard to the percentages of these patients who were regarded by ENT as needing no further management, in all cases this was very high. In all but one project it was 90% or over; the exception being Brown, at 86%.

Table 9.2

ENT actions on patients not cross-referred

	Total not crossed	No further management	Differ on aid only	Dewax only	Further management
Orange			not known		
Red			not known		
Yellow	143	90%	7%	<1%	3%
Green	132	93	2	<1	5
Blue(NH)	198	94	<1	4	2
Blue(PD)	222	94	0	5	1
White	252	98	1	<1	<1
Black	116	97	2	<1	<1
Grey	147	94	0	3	3
Brown	232	86	2	<1	11
Silver	147	93	3	<1	3
Gold	150	99	<1	<1	0
Bronze	134	>99	0	0	<1

9.6.3 Rates of disagreement regarding the fitting of the aid were very low at almost all Centres; the only notable figure being 7% at Yellow. Rates of wax removal were also very low, standing at 1% or less in eight Centres.

9.6.4 The proportions of not-cross-referred patients needing further management were in most cases low, being only 3% or less at 9 out of 11 projects. The two exceptions were Green, at 5%, and Brown, at 11%. These patients are the most critical cases, as they represent instances where the technician could have missed something important.

9.6.5 The figure for Brown is worth further discussion. A good proportion of this (15 cases out of 25) was due to one particular ENT doctor. In particular, this doctor identified a lot of asymmetric losses in need of investigation: 9 of the 15 cases involved this. Querying this result with the Centre themselves, they arranged an experiment whereby the audiograms and histories for these cases were seen and assessed by two ENT consultants and one SR, each working independently.

9.6.6 One consultant felt that further investigation was warranted in just 1 of the 9 cases; the other consultant and the SR did not feel it was necessary in any case. The two consultants and SR also studied another 5 cases of asymmetric loss, originally identified by other doctors: in only 2 cases did any of them feel that the asymmetry was significant. These results highlight the way that professional judgements can differ between ENT doctors. If the findings of the first consultant were to be accepted, the percentage of patients needing further management at this Centre would nearly halve, from 11% down to 6%. If those of the SR were accepted, it would become even lower.

9.7 Technician failures of management as a proportion of all patients, and ratings of severity of failure
(table 9.3)

9.7.1 Those patients who were not cross-referred but who needed further ENT action represent the most important cases of management failure by technicians. By looking at these in relation to the total number of patients seen at each Centre, an overall 'failure rate' for each project can be computed. This rate estimates the percentage of patients who would not receive appropriate management if these were normal DR systems operating without a safety-check element.

9.7.2 It is probable that a number of the management failures are quite serious, while others may not be serious at all. In order to take this into account, Dr S. D. G. Stephens of the Welsh Hearing Institute, who was also adviser to the research, reviewed the pro-formas for each case, and rated each failure as either: a) Potentially Serious (in terms of possible consequences for the patient); b) Moderately Serious; c) Not Serious; or d) Don't Know.

9.7.3 When rating the failures, Dr Stephens was asked to take account of the time that had elapsed between the technician and ENT doctor examinations, and to give a 'don't know' rating in those instances where he felt the failure could have been due to conditions developing in this time interval.

9.7.4 The results are summarized in table 9.3. It can be seen that the rates of technician management failure ranged from 0.0% at Gold, up to 10% at Brown. The latter figure is very exceptional, however, as the next highest is 3.2%, at Green. Six (out of 11) projects had rates of less than 1%. Over all projects combined, the rate was 2.2%, which converts to a technician failure of management in approximately 1 out of every 46 cases.

9.7.5 Many of the failures however, were regarded by Dr Stephens as being not particularly important. Considering only those cases where the failure was rated as potentially serious, rates in many Centres are substantially reduced. This is particularly true of Brown, where just 2 of the 25 cases were rated as potentially serious failures. The highest rate was 4 cases at Grey. Three projects had no potentially serious failures at all, and at 4 others there was just 1. Altogether, there was a total of 15 potentially serious failures of management, which yields a rate across all projects combined of 0.64%; equivalent to 1 in every 156 DR patients. Private dispensers, however, were responsible for 4 of the potentially serious failures, and if these are excluded the rate for NHS technicians alone is 0.56%, or 1 in every 177.

9.7.6 When moderate as well as potentially serious failures are considered, failure rates rise appreciably at only two Centres: Brown (up from .81% to 4.9%); and Green (up from 1.1% to 2.7%). The overall rate of failure including moderates is 1.4%, or around 1 in every 71 patients.

9.7.7 The situation regarding Brown is interesting: in terms of potentially serious failures it compares favourably with the other projects, but a much larger number of moderate failures was also identified. It is the feeling of the evaluators that doctors at Brown (one in particular – see 9.6.5) were more

Table 9.3 Technician management failures (i.e. Patients not crossed but in need of further management)

	Total patients seen	All tech management failures	Potentially serious failure	Moderate failure	Not serious	Don't know	% Failure	% Serious failure	% Serious+ moderate
Orange				not known					
Red				not known					
Yellow	233	4 patients	1	2	1	0	1.7%	.43%	1.3%
Green	186	6	2	3	1	0	3.2	1.1	2.7
Blue(NH)	235	2	1	1	0	0	.85	.43	.85
Blue(PD)	228	2	0	1	1	0	.88	.0	.44
White	337	1	1	0	0	0	.30	.30	.30
Black	148	1	0	1	0	0	.68	.0	.68
Grey	169	5	4	0	1	0	3.0	2.4	2.4
Brown	247	25	2	10	10	3	10.0	.81	4.9
Silver	161	4	3	0	1	0	2.5	1.9	1.9
Gold	266	0	0	0	0	0	.0	.0	.0
Bronze	134	1	1	0	0	0	.75	.75	.75
Overall	2344	51	15	18	15	3	2.2%	.64%	1.4%

cautious than most elsewhere, resulting in a much higher number of technician 'failures'. Dr Stephens rated the great majority of these as 'moderate' or 'not serious'. Doctors at other Centres tended to only want further action on the more serious cases in the first place. Thus it is not that there actually were more cases of failure at Brown, but that many similar cases at other Centres were not regarded to need further management at all.

9.7.8 It is of interest to know whether the rate of management failures by technicians dropped over the course of the projects. In order to examine this, the number of failures at each Centre was computed separately for the first 50% and second 50% of patients seen. This yielded a total of 9 potentially serious failures for the first half of the projects, compared to 6 for the second half. However, 3 of the 9 failures in the first half were due to the private dispenser at Grey, who left approximately half-way through the project. Excluding this Centre, the number of potentially serious failures is 6 in the first half, and 5 in the second. Combining moderate and serious failures, and still excluding Grey, there were 18 such failures in the first half compared to 11 in the second. On a chi-squared test, this difference does not reach significance (chi-square=3.22, df=1, p>0.05). Most of the moderate failures were due to a single Centre, Brown, but excluding this, the difference between halves becomes even lower. Therefore, it must be concluded that the evidence suggests no overall reduction in technician failures of management over the course of the projects.

9.8 Potentially serious management failures and a mixed DR/TR service

9.8.1 Using a sample of over 2,300 DR patients, this study has indicated that technicians at the pilot Centres made potentially serious errors of management – relative to the decisions of their local ENT doctors – in around 1 out of every 156 DR patients (or 1 in 177, excluding the private dispensers). If these were 'normal' DR systems, none of these patients would have been seen by an ENT doctor, and they might therefore have missed out on important management; whereas – on the basis of the ENT safety-check – if they had come through TR they would have been picked up. These cases can therefore be thought of as representing additional potentially serious failures which result from operating Direct Referral (i.e. additional to any failures which might occur under an exclusively TR system).

9.8.2 As a rule, Centres which run DR do so alongside a TR service (since not all patients are suitable for DR). Therefore it is relevant to ask what these additional failures amount to as a proportion of all hearing aid patients from both systems combined. It will be seen in a later section (21.1) that towards the end of the pilot projects around 36% of all patients fitted with hearing aids were coming through DR, and 64% through TR. On this basis, the rate of additional potentially serious failures under a mixed DR/TR service – compared to TR operating on its own – is around 1 in every 430 patients seen.

9.8.3 There is evidence, however, that the ENT safety-checks of DR patients under the pilot projects were in some cases performed to a lower standard than many normal ENT clinic examinations, and that the rates of technician failures – as detected by ENT doctors – reported in this chapter may be slightly lower than they would have been if this were not the case. This evidence, together with rates estimated on a different basis plus a much fuller discussion of the findings and their implications, appears in the next chapter, which is concerned with the medical examinations of samples of patients by external specialists.

9.9 The types of technician management failure
(table 9.4)

9.9.1 By far the most common condition amongst the cases that technicians failed on was asymmetric loss: this featured in 19 of the total of 51 cases, and 9 of the 15 serious cases. There were many instances, however, where a technician noted that asymmetric loss was present, but did not cross-referred.

Table 9.4
Details of management failures by technicians (all centres)

Potentially serious technician failures

ENT management	Reasons for management	Relevant technician findings
Treatment	Cholesteatoma	
Investigate	Asymmetric loss	Noted by technician
Investigate	Asymmetric loss	Noted by technician
Investigate	Fluctuating asymmetric loss	
Investigate	Asymmetric loss	
Investigate	Asymmetric loss	
Investigate	Asymmetric loss	Noted by technician
Investigate	Unilateral sudden deafness	Noted as investigated in 1986
Investigate	Vertigo	Noted as being treated by GP
Investigate	Solar keratosis, right ear	
Review	Asymmetric loss	Noted by technician
Review	Noise exposure/attic pocket	Tech noted mixed loss
Review	Asymmetric loss	
Review	Deep right attic pocket	
Refer on	Solar keratosis right pinna, referred to dermatologist	

Moderately serious technician failures

ENT management	Reasons for management	Relevant technician findings
Treatment	Wart in right ear canal	
Treatment	Otitis external, right ear	
Treatment+Review	Otitis external (worse in ear fitted)	
Treatment	Middle ear effusion (developed since fitting)	
Investigate	Asymmetric loss	
Investigate	Asymmetric loss	
Investigate	Asymmetric loss	
Investigate	Conductive loss	
Investigate	Husky voice	
Investigate	Vertigo and tinnitus	Tech noted tinnitus
Investigate	Deviated nasal septum and rhinitis	
Investigate	Perf+asym (patient refused invest)	Tech noted asym loss
Investigate	Thyroid swelling	
Review	Perforation	Noted by technician
Review	Mastoid	
Review	Otosclerosis/asymmetric loss	

| Review | Advice on tinnitus needed | |
| Review | Otosclerosis | Tech noted conductive loss |

Not serious technician failures

ENT management	Reasons for management	Relevant technician findings
Investigate	Asymmetric loss	
Investigate	Asymmetric loss	
Investigate	Asymmetric loss	
Investigate	Asymmetric loss	
Investigate	Poor discrimination/vertigo	
Investigate	Conductive loss (patient refused invest)	Tech noted asym loss
Investigate	Bilateral loss in young person (age 34)	
Review	Asymmetric loss	
Review	Patient does not want aid at present	
Review	Aid not required at present	Tech also advised review
Review	Aid not required at present	
Review	Aid not required at present	
Review	Repeat audio (reason not given)	
Critical of Tech	Aid fitted to ear blocked with wax	
Critical of Tech	Aid fitted to ear blocked with wax	

Don't know

ENT management	Reasons for management	Relevant technician findings
Investigate	Tinnitus, left ear	
Review	Check hearing isn't deteriorating	
Refer on	Refer to hearing therapist if problems persist	

9.9.2 The fact that nearly two-thirds of serious failures were cases of asymmetrical loss is a significant finding. In particular, it should not be too difficult to reduce these numbers by adjusting technician practice. Unfortunately, the audiograms for these patients are not available, and so it is not known whether the cases fail the TTSA criteria for significant asymmetry, or whether the technicians did not follow the criteria properly. Nevertheless, such failures could be reduced in future either by modifying the criteria, or – if they are considered adequate as they stand – by ensuring that technicians obey them to the letter.

9.9.3 In the next chapter we will see strong evidence of a wide disparity between ENT doctors regarding the management of asymmetrical losses. It is our opinion that the reason why technicians as a group failed to cross-refer a substantial number of these was largely because they tried to follow local practice, which often did not adhere to set rules and could vary between doctors within the same department, rather than sticking to a fixed criteria.

9.9.4 The other serious management failures involved two instances of attic retraction pocket, two solar keratoses, one cases of vertigo, and a cholesteatoma. In two cases the technician identified the condition but did not refer to ENT because it had either been investigated in the past or was under GP treatment. However, Dr Stephens felt that the pathology was so serious that the technician should nevertheless have cross-referred.

9.9.5 Also of interest is the fact that of a total of 4 cases of cholesteatoma picked up by ENT doctors across all Centres over the pilot period, technicians detected and cross-referred 3.

9.9.6 Finally, a comment is appropriate regarding non-otological medical conditions that may be associated with hearing loss, most notably vascular and metabolic disorders and drug-induced ototoxicity (see 9.2.3, above). Out of the total 51 cases of technician management failure, there were just 3 where the ENT doctor had noted anything falling into this category, all vascular problems. However, in every case the condition was already under treatment and was not part of the reason for deciding on further management. This finding is not surprising, as it seems unlikely that the safety-check doctors checked to see if any such (undiagnosed) conditions were present.

9.10 Serious management failures and technician grade

9.10.1 With regard to the grades of technicians who committed serious management failures, these were broadly spread: 4 failures were by private dispensers; 2 involved technicians of MTO5; 1 was by an MTO4; 6 by MTO3's; and 2 by MTO2's. Although MTO3's are the single largest category, these technicians saw the largest number of patients (50% of the total), and their rate of failures is actually lower than for the other grades.

9.10.2 Of the 4 serious failures by private dispensers, 3 of these were committed by the same person. Other aspects of the performance of the dispensers are discussed in section 18.

9.10.3 With regard to the failures by NHS technicians, there was no suggestion that these were due to a few particular individuals. Quite the reverse in fact, as the 11 serious failures here involved 10 different technicians across 8 different Centres.

10 Patient Safety: Medical Examinations by External Specialists

10.1 Introduction

10.1.1 Chapter nine examined the safety of the Direct Referral procedures in terms of technician performance relative to clinical decisions made by their own ENT doctors. It is possible however, that ENT doctors themselves at times make errors of judgement. A complete examination of patient safety needs to take this factor into account. In order to do this, the research project engaged the help of two ENT specialists, both of high standing, who were independent of any of the pilot Centres. The two 'External Specialists' between them visited 9 of the 12 Centres between September 1991 and January 1992, and they made medical examinations on totals of 239 DR patients and 216 TR patients. The results of these examinations were then used to assess the performance of the technicians and local ENT doctors who had examined the patients previously. The purpose of this exercise was to provide measures of patient safety under the two referral systems which would be based on external, expert, judgement.

10.1.2 Before going into the details of the methodology used in this exercise, a brief summary is given below to aid clarity. The steps of the methodology are also presented as a flow diagram in figure 10.1.

10.1.3 *Summary of Methodology.* All of the patients seen by the external specialists (with very few exceptions) had been examined previously by a technician and local ENT doctor (at the safety-check) if they were DRs, or by just a local ENT doctor if TRs (at a routine ENT clinic). When the external specialist visits were complete, the results for patients whom they considered to need more management than just the fitting of a hearing aid (or simple dewax) were selected out. Two 'Expert Assessors' then compared the details of the previous technician and/or ENT doctor examinations for these cases with the findings of the specialists, using the latter as the 'Gold Standard'. Each expert made independent assessments of the severity of any medical conditions present, and gave pass/fail ratings to the technician's and/or local doctor's diagnosis and management of each patient.

10.2 Methodology – external specialist examinations

10.2.1 The specialist examinations were done such that the specialists were kept blind as to which patients were TR and which DR, and overall there were only two instances where they discovered the fact – from inadvertent comments by the patients involved. They were also kept blind – as far as practically possible – to the management decisions made by the technician

Figure 10.1

Flow diagram illustrating
methodology of safety
experiment

Two external ENT specialists conduct examinations on samples of DR and TR patients at pilot Centres. One specialist visits 4 Centres, and the other 5. The specialists are kept blind as to which patients are DR and which TR. They are also blind to the findings of the technicians and/or ENT doctors who had previously examined the patients. Totals of 239 DR and 216 TR patients are examined

Those cases where the specialists wanted more management than just hearing aid fitting or simple dewax are selected out. These comprise 26 DR and 54 TR patients The following steps are undertaken for these cases only

Two 'Experts' make independent assessments based on the clinical findings for each of these patients. Using the specialists' findings as the 'gold standard', for each patient the two experts assess: (a) The severity of any ear conditions and (b) The technician's and/or ENT doctor's diagnosis and management of the patient

Analysis of resulting data

and local ENT doctor who had previously seen each patient (except for the fact that all patients had been fitted with hearing aids). These conditions were imposed in order to prevent knowledge of the route or previous management from influencing the decisions made by the specialists themselves.

10.2.2 The specialists were not given access to hospital notes, as these would have revealed the route of provision and previous management. Instead, each patient's audiogram was provided, together with any other test results that the technician or ENT doctor had access to when they examined the patient. In very few cases was there anything other than the audiogram. Centres were also asked to write down any other information about the patient they felt the specialist should be aware of (e.g. medication), provided this did not violate the test conditions.

10.2.3 There was inevitably an interval of time between the specialists seeing the patients and their previous examinations, either by a technician or an ENT doctor. To minimise the effect of this it was stipulated that all patients should have been fitted not more than two months previous. A number of Centres found it difficult to find the required number of patients (willing to attend) within this time-span, and so the criteria was stretched for these Centres in order to reach the quota. The time-span limitation had an added advantage of giving Centres little room to be selective about the patients invited to attend, thus ensuring that the samples would be fairly random (though self-selected).

10.2.4 Although it was intended that all of the DR patients should have had their safety-check prior to being seen by a specialist, there were a few occasions where this had not happened, and the safety-check was conducted after the specialist's examination. There were two such instances amongst those cases that specialists felt needed more management than just the hearing aid. It does not appear, however, that the ENT doctors involved came to know of the specialist's findings, as in neither case did they pick up the condition for which management was required.

10.3 Methodology – involvement of independent expert assessors

10.3.1 Comparison of the specialist findings and management decisions with those of local technicians and ENT doctors was a critical part of the exercise. To make the comparisons, the aid of two independent expert assessors was engaged. One expert was Dr S D G Stephens, of the Welsh Hearing Institute, who was also acting as an advisor to the research project. The other expert was Mr R Ramsden, consultant ENT surgeon, of Manchester. Mr Ramsden specialises in acoustic neuroma, which was very valuable as this condition causes great concern with regard to safety of the DR procedure.

10.3.2 The intention was that the findings of the specialists would be used as the 'Gold Standard' against which the previous examinations would be compared. Therefore, cases where the specialists did not suggest any management other than an aid were assumed to present nothing of clinical significance, and were not assessed by the expert assessors. There were a total of 26 DR cases and 54 TR cases which the specialists had identified as in need of further management.

10.3.3 Before the experts could assess the TR cases however, copies of notes in each patient's hospital file about previous ENT examinations and management had to be obtained. Under NHS rules of confidentiality, the permission of each patient was required before access to the notes could be given. In most cases this was obtained by post. Permission was received, and ENT notes obtained, for 49 of the 54 cases. Therefore each expert independently assessed the 26 DR cases requiring further management, and the 49 TR cases for which notes were available.

10.3.4 Each expert was supplied with copies of the examinations made by the specialist, the technician (DR cases only), and the ENT doctor, together with each patient's audiogram and any other audiological test results which were available to previous examiners. Important background information about each patient, such as age and relevant previous medical history, was also provided. The experts were then asked to rate a) the diagnosis and b) the management, that had been decided upon by the technician and ENT doctor. Diagnosis and management were each rated as either Pass, Fail, or Don't Know.

10.3.5 The term 'diagnosis' is used in a loose way here, and refers more to the identification of clinically significant factors (e.g. asymmetric loss, discharging ears), than it does to making a specific diagnosis of what any underlying pathology might be. For simplicity, the term 'diagnosis' is used to refer to the findings of technicians as well as those of doctors.

10.3.6 In the event, the ratings given by the experts to diagnosis performance were the same as those for management in the great majority of cases (i.e. they tended to be either both 'pass' or both 'fail'). Therefore in order to simplify the presentation of results, the findings for diagnosis are not discussed below. However, the results are summarized in the tables.

10.3.7 When rating management, the experts were asked to make the ratings *according to their own standards*. That is, they were not required to accept the specialist's decision on management as absolute. Thus, there were a few cases where one or both experts found themselves in agreement with the local doctor rather than with the specialist.

10.3.8 In addition to diagnosis and management, each expert was asked to rate the *potential* severity of any consequences for the patient if they did not receive appropriate management for any identified conditions (excluding simple age-related hearing loss). Potential severity was rated as either 'Serious (for the patient)', 'Moderately Serious', 'Not Serious', or 'Don't Know'. It must be emphasised that the experts were only rating the *potential* severity of any conditions: it was of-course impossible to know what any actual consequences would be. Also, in most cases the conditions identified were signs (e.g. asymmetrical hearing loss) of possible disease, but there may in fact have been no actual underlying pathology.

10.3.9 In making their ratings, the experts were asked to take into account the time that had elapsed between examinations. In particular, where there were disagreements, whether these could have been due to conditions developing or abating during this interval.

10.4 Methodology – expert assessment of technician cross-referral performance

10.4.1 In addition to rating diagnosis and management, Dr Stephens also assessed each DR case as to whether the technician should or should not have cross-referred to an ENT doctor. This was irrespective of whether he considered the patient to display any conditions of real concern: some conditions need a doctors opinion if only to be passed as non-significant.

10.4.2 It is convenient to deal with the results of this exercise here, before getting on to the more complex analysis of management performance. Dr Stephens considered 23% of the DR sample to require cross-referral, and 77% not to do so. Technicians in fact crossed only half (51%) of those thought to require cross-referral. Over the sample as a whole, technicians took the correct action in 83% of cases; failed to cross 11%; and unnecessarily cross-referred 6%.

10.5 Results – the findings of the external specialists
(tables 10.1 to 10.3)

10.5.1 The principal actions that the specialists could decide upon were: a) Appropriate to fit Hearing Aid; b) Further investigation required; c) Medical intervention required; and d) Patient needs reviewing again at later date. For the purposes of analysis, the last three categories are frequently grouped together under the heading 'further management needed'. There were also a very small number of patients who required wax removal only – these have not been included in the group needing further management, except in three instances where special circumstances were present (they are treated as 'reviews').

10.5.2 *DR Patients.* Of the 239 DR patients seen by the specialists, in 89% of cases the only management needed was aid fitting ('on trial' in some instances). 8% of patients (20 in total) were considered to also need further investigation or medical treatment, and the remaining 3% (6 patients) required a review at a later date.

10.5.3 At all Centres bar one the percentage of DR patients needing further management was low, never more than 12%. The exception to this had a much higher figure, 36%. This Centre alone accounts for 38% of all DR patients needing further management.

10.5.4 It is of interest to note that local ENT doctors themselves had wanted further action in only 3 of the 26 cases identified by specialists (1 investigation and 2 reviews). This demonstrates that a substantial gulf existed between local standards and those used by the specialists when making their examinations.

10.5.5 *TR Patients.* Of the 216 TR patients some 75% only required hearing aid fitting. In another 21% (46 cases) the specialists advised further investigation or treatment in addition to aid fitting; and in the other 5% (8 cases) fitting plus review was required. The total proportion of TR patients needing further action was just over double the proportion of DR patients: 25% compared to 11%. A difference in proportions is to be expected given that GPs are supposed to select 'clean' patients for DR – indeed, it would be rather worrying if there were no difference.

10.5.6 The numbers of TRs needing action were quite variable from one Centre to another. At one place no TR cases were found to require further management, but there were 5 Centres where it was over 30%. The highest proportion anywhere was 37%.

10.5.7 The reasons for requiring further management are listed for each individual DR and TR case in tables 10.2 and 10.3. Also appearing in these tables are the ratings made by the expert assessors of the severity of the conditions presented, and also the ratings of the management performance of technicians and ENT doctors.

10.6 Results – expert assessments of severity of patients' conditions (tables 10.1 to 10.3)

10.6.1 *DR patients*. Of the 26 DR patients that (according to the specialists) required further management, the first expert rated 10 cases as 'serious or potentially serious (if not managed)', 5 as moderately serious, and 11 as not serious. The corresponding figures for the second expert were 15, 4, and 7, respectively.

10.6.2 Overall, the experts gave the same rating in only 50% of the cases. However, most of the disagreement was between adjacent categories; that is, between 'serious' and 'moderate', and 'moderate' and 'not serious'. The amount of agreement including these rises to 77%. This still leaves 6 cases (23%) which one expert rated as potentially serious and the other as not serious.

10.6.3 Under the assumption that none of the cases considered to need no further management (and hence not assessed by the experts) had significant pathology, the first expert's assessments suggest that 4.2% of DR patients attend with a potentially serious condition (i.e. 10 out of 239). The corresponding figure for the second expert is 6.3% (15 out of 239).

10.6.4 By combining the results for the two experts it is possible to put approximate lower and upper bounds on the 'true' percentage attending with a potentially serious condition. There were 8 cases rated potentially serious by *both* experts, and this suggests a lower bound of 3.3%. However, 17 cases were rated potentially serious by *at least one* expert, which yields an upper bound of 7.1%.

10.6.5 *TR patients*. The first expert rated 17 of the 49 TR patients as exhibiting potentially serious conditions, 16 as moderate, and 16 as not serious. Figures for the second expert were 23, 4, and 22 respectively. The principal difference between the experts was that the second made far less use of the 'moderate' category.

10.6.6 Agreement between the experts was very much on a par with that found for DR patients. There was complete agreement in 51% of cases, and agreement within one category ran at 84%. In all, there were 8 cases (16%) which one expert rated as potentially serious and the other as not serious.

10.6.7 The figures yield rates of potentially serious conditions amongst TR patients of 8.1% (17 out of 211) and 10.9% (23 out of 211) for each expert respectively. 12 cases were rated potentially serious by *both*, while 28 were so rated by *at least one*. These suggest lower and upper bounds on the real percentage of 5.7% and 13.3%. These rates are just under double those for DR patients, and concur with the previous finding that the proportion needing further management was also about double.

Table 10.1
Summary of external
specialist assessments

DR patients – management decisions by external specialists

Action	Freq	%
Fit Aid Only (in some cases on trial)	213	89
Further Investigation/Medical Intervention	20	8
Review again at later date	6	3

Total cases needing further management = 26 out of 239

Expert assessments of potential severity of DR patient conditions

	Pot. serious	Moderate	Not serious	Don't know
First Expert	10	5	11	0
Second Expert	15	4	7	0

Total cases assessed = 26

Cross-tabulation of severity assessments on DR patients

		EXPERT 2		
		Pot. serious	Moderate	Not serious
	Pot. serious	8	1	1
EXPERT 1	Moderate	2	1	2
	Not serious	5	2	4

Agreement = 50%   Agreement within one category = 77%

TR patients – management decisions by external specialists

Action	Freq	%
Fit Aid Only (in some cases on trial)	162	75
Further Investigation/Medical Intervention	46	21
Review again at later date	8	5

Total cases needing further management = 54 out of 216

Expert assessments of potential severity of TR patient conditions

	Pot. serious	Moderate	Not serious	Don't know
First Expert	17	16	16	0
Second Expert	23	4	22	0

Total cases assessed = 49 (ENT notes not available for 5)

Cross-tabulation of severity assessments on TR patients

		EXPERT 2		
		Pot. serious	Moderate	Not serious
	Pot.serious	12	1	4
EXPERT 1	Moderate	7	2	7
	Not serious	4	1	11

Agreement = 51%   Agreement within one category = 84%

Table 10.2 DR cases where external specialists indicated that further management was needed

Reason for action	Techs action	ENT action	Severity of condition		Technician management		ENT management	
			Expert 1	Expert 2	Expert 1	Expert 2	Expert 1	Expert 2
CASES NEEDING INVESTIGATION/TREATMENT								
1. Rodent Ulcer	FIT	FIT	SERIOUS	SERIOUS	FAIL	FAIL	FAIL	FAIL
2. Asymmetry+Tinnitus	FIT	FIT	SERIOUS	SERIOUS	FAIL	FAIL	FAIL	FAIL
3. Asymmetry+Conductive loss+Tinn	FIT	DK	SERIOUS	SERIOUS	FAIL	FAIL	DK	DK
4. Asymmetry+Vertigo	FIT	DK	SERIOUS	SERIOUS	FAIL	FAIL	DK	DK
5. Fluid+Possible Tumour	CROSS	FIT	SERIOUS	SERIOUS	PASS	PASS	FAIL	FAIL
6. Asymmetry+voice problem	CROSS	FIT	SERIOUS	SERIOUS	PASS	PASS	FAIL	FAIL
7. Mixed Loss+Otitis+Indrawn drum	CROSS	INVEST	SERIOUS	SERIOUS	PASS	PASS	FAIL	FAIL
8. Asymmetry+Tinnitus	CROSS	FIT	SERIOUS	SERIOUS	PASS	PASS	PASS	PASS
9. Asymmetry (completely dead ear)	CROSS	FIT	SERIOUS	MOD	PASS	PASS	PASS	PASS
10. Asym+Cond+Fluid in middle ear	CROSS	FIT	MOD	SERIOUS	PASS	PASS	FAIL	FAIL
11. Active discharge+Hard wax	CROSS	REVIEW	MOD	SERIOUS	PASS	PASS	PASS	PASS
12. Asymmetric Loss	CROSS	FIT	MOD	MOD	PASS	PASS	FAIL	FAIL
13. Very deaf for age	FIT	FIT	MOD	NS	PASS	DK	PASS	FAIL
14. Conductive loss+Unusual audio	FIT	FIT	NS	SERIOUS	FAIL	FAIL	FAIL	FAIL
15. Possibly underlying CSOM	FIT	FIT	NS	SERIOUS	FAIL	FAIL	FAIL	PASS
16. Hard wax blocking ears	FIT	FIT	NS	SERIOUS	FAIL	PASS	FAIL	PASS
17. Asymmetry+Tinnitus+Sudden Onset	DK	FIT	NS	SERIOUS	DK	DK	FAIL	FAIL
18. Otosclerosis+sound distortion	CROSS	FIT	NS	SERIOUS	PASS	PASS	FAIL	PASS
19. May have URTI	FIT	DK	NS	MOD	FAIL	FAIL	DK	DK
20. Mixed deafness	CROSS	REVIEW	NS	NS	PASS	PASS	FAIL	PASS
CASES NEEDING A REVIEW								
21. Wax in ear altered by surgery	FIT	FIT	SERIOUS	NS	FAIL	PASS	DK	FAIL
22. Otitis Externa	CROSS	FIT	MOD	MOD	PASS	PASS	PASS	DK
23. Unusual audiogram	CROSS	FIT	NS	MOD	PASS	PASS	FAIL	FAIL
24. Improved diagnosis needed	FIT	FIT	NS	NS	FAIL	FAIL	FAIL	FAIL
25. Loss may be progressive	FIT	FIT	NS	NS	FAIL	PASS	FAIL	PASS
26. Unusual audiogram	FIT	FIT	NS	NS	PASS	PASS	PASS	PASS

58

Table 10.3 TR cases where specialists wanted further management

Case	Reason for action	Severity of condition Expert 1	Expert 2	ENT management Expert 1	Expert 2
CASES NEEDING INVESTIGATION/TREATMENT					
1.	Possible Cholesteatoma	SERIOUS	SERIOUS	FAIL	FAIL
2.	Asymmetric loss	SERIOUS	SERIOUS	FAIL	FAIL
3.	Asymmetric loss	SERIOUS	SERIOUS	FAIL	FAIL
4.	Asymmetric loss	SERIOUS	SERIOUS	FAIL	FAIL
5.	Asymmetric loss	SERIOUS	SERIOUS	FAIL	FAIL
6.	Asymmetric loss	SERIOUS	SERIOUS	PASS	FAIL
7.	Asymmetric loss – Possible neuroma	SERIOUS	SERIOUS	FAIL	FAIL
8.	Asymmetric loss+Tinnitus	SERIOUS	SERIOUS	PASS	PASS
9.	Tumour Right Auditory Meatus	SERIOUS	SERIOUS	PASS	PASS
10.	Asymmetric loss+Tinnitus	SERIOUS	SERIOUS	PASS	PASS
11.	Asymmetric loss+Tinnitus	SERIOUS	SERIOUS	PASS	PASS
12.	Asym – Menière's disease	SERIOUS	SERIOUS	PASS	PASS
13.	Asymmetric loss	SERIOUS	MOD	PASS	FAIL
14.	Asymmetric loss	SERIOUS	NS	FAIL	PASS
15.	Pain left ear+Tinnitus	SERIOUS	NS	FAIL	PASS
16.	Asymmetric loss	SERIOUS	NS	FAIL	PASS
17.	Carcinoma of the breast (SEE A)	SERIOUS	NS	FAIL	PASS
18.	Asymmetric loss	MOD	SERIOUS	FAIL	FAIL
19.	Feeling of blockage in ear	MOD	SERIOUS	FAIL	FAIL
20.	Asymmetric loss	MOD	SERIOUS	PASS	FAIL
21.	Pain right ear, blood in mouth	MOD	SERIOUS	PASS	DK
22.	CSOM+Perforation	MOD	SERIOUS	PASS	PASS
23.	Conductive loss – Bilateral CSOM	MOD	SERIOUS	PASS	PASS
24.	Severe deafness	MOD	MOD	FAIL	FAIL
25.	Conductive loss+Perforation	MOD	MOD	PASS	PASS
26.	Asymmetric loss+Conductive loss	MOD	NS	FAIL	PASS
27.	Conductive loss – Otosclerosis?	MOD	NS	PASS	PASS
28.	Chronic Otitis+Perforation	MOD	NS	PASS	PASS
29.	Chronic ear infection	MOD	NS	PASS	PASS
30.	Conductive loss+Aid in wrong ear?	MOD	NS	PASS	PASS
31.	Asymmetric loss+Conductive loss	MOD	NS	PASS	PASS
32.	Conductive loss – Bilateral CSOM	NS	SERIOUS	PASS	FAIL
33.	Very deaf for age+Cond loss	NS	SERIOUS	FAIL	FAIL
34.	Mixed loss+Bilateral CSOM+Perf	NS	SERIOUS	PASS	PASS
35.	Very deaf for age	NS	SERIOUS	PASS	FAIL
36.	Unusual audiogram	NS	MOD	PASS	FAIL
37.	Otosclerosis	NS	NS	PASS	PASS
38.	Sinus infection	NS	NS	PASS	FAIL
39.	Very deaf for age	NS	NS	PASS	PASS
40.	Conductive loss – Aid in wrong ear?	NS	NS	PASS	PASS
41.	Severe loss	NS	NS	PASS	PASS
42.	Severe loss	NS	NS	PASS	PASS
CASES NEEDING A REVIEW					
43.	Discharging ears	MOD	SERIOUS	PASS	PASS
44.	Tinnitus advice needed	MOD	NS	PASS	PASS
45.	Advice on balance problem	NS	NS	PASS	PASS
46.	Tinnitus	NS	NS	PASS	PASS
47.	Hearing may be deteriorating	NS	NS	PASS	PASS
48.	Unusual history	NS	NS	PASS	PASS
49.	Dewax under microscope	NS	NS	PASS	PASS

A)   The second expert excluded this from his rating of severity.

10.7 Results – expert assessments of patient management
(tables 10.4 to 10.5)

10.7.1 The results of the expert assessments of patient management will be examined in three different ways. Firstly, the performance of technicians and doctors with respect to their management of patients will be examined. Secondly, the performance of the DR and TR *systems* of provision will be compared. Thirdly, examination will be made of the relative performance of *a mixture of DR and TR systems* – as is the usual situation in practice – compared to an exclusively TR service.

Table 10.4

Expert assessments of technician and doctor performance

DR patients – ratings of diagnosis

		Pass	Fail	Don't know
TECHNICIANS	Expert 1	15	11	0
	Expert 2	18	7	1
ENT DOCTORS	Expert 1	11	11	4
	Expert 2	11	11	4

DR patients – rating of management

		Pass	Fail	Don't know
TECHNICIANS	Expert 1	14	11	1
	Expert 2	16	8	2
ENT DOCTORS	Expert 1	5	17	4
	Expert 2	9	13	4

DR patients – potential severity of management failures

		Pot. serious	Mod	NS
TECHNICIANS	Expert 1	5	0	6
	Expert 2	6	1	1
ENT DOCTORS	Expert 1	6	2	9
	Expert 2	8	2	3

TR patients – ratings of ENT diagnosis

	Pass	Fail	Don't know
Expert 1	32	16	1
Expert 2	33	16	0

TR patients – rating of ENT management

	Pass	Fail	Don't know
Expert 1	34	15	0
Expert 2	31	17	1

TR patients – potential severity of management failures

	Pot. serious	Moderate	Not serious
Expert 1	10	4	1
Expert 2	13	3	1

Table 10.5

Comparison of expert assessments

DR patients: cross-tabulation of diagnosis ratings – technicians

		EXPERT 2		
		Pass	Fail	Don't know
EXPERT 1	Pass	13	1	1
	Fail	5	6	0
	Don't know	0	0	0

Agreement = 76%   Kappa = 0.49   (don't knows excluded)

DR patients: cross-tabulation of diagnosis ratings – ENT doctors

		EXPERT 2		
		Pass	Fail	Don't know
EXPERT 1	Pass	8	2	1
	Fail	3	8	0
	Don't know	0	1	3

Agreement = 76%   Kappa = 0.53   (don't knows excluded)

DR patients: cross-tabulation of management ratings – technicians

		EXPERT 2		
		Pass	Fail	Don't know
EXPERT 1	Pass	13	0	1
	Fail	3	8	0
	Don't know	0	0	1

Agreement = 88%   Kappa = 0.75   (don't knows excluded)

DR patients: cross-tabulation of management ratings – doctors

		EXPERT 2		
		Pass	Fail	Don't know
EXPERT 1	Pass	3	1	1
	Fail	6	11	0
	Don't know	0	1	3

Agreement = 67%   Kappa = 0.28   (don't knows excluded)

TR patients: cross-tabulation of diagnosis ratings – doctors

		EXPERT 2		
		Pass	Fail	Don't know
EXPERT 1	Pass	28	4	0
	Fail	5	11	0
	Don't know	0	1	0

Agreement = 81%   Kappa = 0.57   (Don't Knows excluded)

TR patients: cross-tabulation of management ratings – doctors

		EXPERT 2		
		Pass	Fail	Don't know
EXPERT 1	Pass	26	7	1
	Fail	5	10	0
	Don't know	0	0	0

Agreement = 75%   Kappa = 0.44   (Don't Knows excluded)

10.7.2 *Levels of agreement between the experts.* To simplify the subsequent presentation of results, it is useful to deal first with the question of how much the experts agreed in their assessments. Percentage agreement figures have been computed for the ratings of diagnosis and management for doctors seeing TR patients, and for both doctors and technicians seeing DR patients (table 10.5). Agreement was at 75% or above for 5 out of the 6 measures. The exception was the ratings of management for doctors seeing DR patients, where the two experts agreed just 67% of the time (i.e. in one-third of cases one expert passed the management while the other failed it).

10.7.3 Cohen's kappa has been computed in each case. A value of kappa of 0.6 or above is generally taken as indicating an acceptable level of agreement (Hartmann, 1977). Only one of the 6 kappa values was above 0.6, with most being around the 0.5 level, indicating that the general level of agreement between experts was rather low. This finding concurs with observations made elsewhere in this report about the considerable variety of professional opinion in this field.

10.7.4 Despite the above, however, it will be seen in the presentation of results that the overall conclusions reached are the same irrespective of whichever set of expert ratings are used.

10.7.5 *Treatment of missing data.* For a few patients data was incomplete, either because the technician or ENT pro-forma was missing or because one or the other expert gave a 'don't know' rating. There was, in fact, slightly more missing data from doctors than from technicians. In order to maintain as large a sample as possible, each result presented below is based upon as many complete cases as possible, which means that sample sizes vary between experts, and between technicians and doctors. However, parallel analyses have been run excluding incomplete cases across the board, and while differing from the results presented in small details, the basic findings and general conclusions were not altered.

10.8 Results – technician and doctor performance with respect to patient management
(table 10.6)

10.8.1 Before considering the results with respect to patient management, it is important to make the point that technician management and doctor management are not equivalent things. With technicians, 'management' principally refers to whether patients were appropriately cross-referred to ENT; whereas for doctors it refers to whether everything appropriate was done to ensure that significant treatable pathology did not go undetected. However, it is probably easier to say that a patient shows signs that an ENT doctor should look at, than it is for an ENT doctor to say whether those signs indicate anything significant. For this reason no direct comparison is made between the performance rates of technicians and doctors. Although deciding on appropriate ENT management can be complex, it should be noted that in the present study almost all instances where the experts' disagreed with the local ENT management were cases where the former felt that some form of further investigation was required, whereas the latter had simply discharged the patient. Therefore, the disagreements presented here are not over

Table 10.6

Management performance
of technicians and doctors

Management of pathology when present–all cases needing management

		No. of passes	No. needing management	Pass rate
DR – TECHS	Expert 1	14	25	56%
	Expert 2	16	24	67%
DR – DOCS	Expert 1	5	22	23%
	Expert 2	9	22	41%
TR – DOCS	Expert 1	34	49	69%
	Expert 2	31	48	65%

Management of pathology when present – potentially serious cases only

		No. of passes	No. serious cases	Pass rate
DR – TECHS	Expert 1	5	10	50%
	Expert 2	8	14	57%
DR – DOCS	Expert 1	1	7	14%
	Expert 2	5	13	38%
TR – DOCS	Expert 1	7	17	41%
	Expert 2	9	22	41%

Overall rates of failures of management

		No. of fails	Total cases	Failure rate
DR – TECHS	Expert 1	11	238	4.6%
	Expert 2	8	237	3.4%
DR – DOCS	Expert 1	17	235	7.2%
	Expert 2	13	235	5.5%
TR – DOCS	Expert 1	15	211	7.1%
	Expert 2	17	210	8.1%

Overall rates of potentially serious failures of management

		Pot. serious fails	Total cases	Failure rate
DR – TECHS	Expert 1	5	238	2.1%
	Expert 2	6	237	2.5%
DR – DOCS	Expert 1	6	235	2.6%
	Expert 2	8	235	3.4%
TR – DOCS	Expert 1	10	211	4.7%
	Expert 2	13	210	6.2%

'nuances' of the management undertaken, but do represent substantive differences.

10.8.2 It has been explained that the intention was to treat the findings of the external specialists (and therefore the consequent expert assessments) as a 'Gold Standard' against which the performance of technicians and local doctors would be measured. However, it has also been noted that a considerable degree of difference of opinion was found between the two experts themselves, and that this echoed the generally wide variation in professional opinion evident in this field. This factor makes any 'Gold Standard' one sets somewhat arbitrary. Nevertheless, it is necessary to have a standard or it becomes impossible to make any judgement at all. This study has tried to ensure that the standard it uses – while undoubtedly to some degree arbitrary – was at least set by professionals with a widely acknowledged standing in the field. It is nonetheless important to bear in mind that the results presented in this and subsequent sections are measured relative to this standard, and do not have the status of 'absolute' findings. In order to avoid the use of terms which might mislead on this point (such as 'success rate'), the phrase 'MPE rate', meaning 'Management Passed by the Expert(s)', is frequently used below when presenting results.

10.8.3 *Technician Management of DR Patients.* Of those DR patients considered to require some form of further management (other than a hearing aid), the first expert agreed with the technician's management in 14 out of 25 instances (56%). The corresponding figure for the second expert was 16 out of 24 (67%). These results yield an average rate of technician management passed by the experts (MPE rate) *when management other than an aid is required* of 61%.

10.8.4 Expressed as a rate across all patients seen, the results indicate that – in the view of the experts - technicians appropriately managed 97.5% of all DR patients (not taking into account unnecessary cross-referrals).

10.8.5 *Technician Management of Potentially Serious Conditions.* Many of the conditions presented by patients and considered to need further management were rated as being either 'not serious' or of only 'moderate' severity by the expert assessors. The cases of most concern are those that were assessed as being of a 'potentially serious' nature. Therefore these are subjected to a separate analysis below.

10.8.6 The first expert considered 10 DR patients to present potentially serious conditions, of which 5 (50%) were cross-referred to ENT by the technician. The second expert regarded 14 DR cases to be of a potentially serious nature, 8 (57%) of which were cross-referred. Averaging the results for the two experts suggests an MPE rate for potentially serious conditions *when present* of 54%. There were 4 cases which both experts agreed were potentially serious technician failures.

10.8.7 Expressed as a rate over all DR patients, potentially serious failures by technicians ran at an average of 2.3% (i.e. according to the experts, around 1 in every 43 DR patients would have potentially serious pathology that a technician would miss).

10.8.8 *Doctor Management of DR Patients.* According to expert 1, local ENT doctors appropriately managed 5 out of 22 DR patients (23%) who were in need of further management; and on expert 2's findings it was 9 out of 22 (41%). This suggests an average MPE rate of 32%.

10.8.9 With regard to potentially serious cases only, the first expert considered just 1 out of a total of 7 patients to have been correctly managed by local doctors (the other six were discharged with no action other than hearing aid fitting). Expert 2 regarded 5 out of 13 potentially serious cases as appropriately managed (38%). The average MPE rate in this case is therefore 26%.

10.8.10 *Doctor Management of TR Patients.* Turning now to the sample of TR patients, we find considerably less disagreement between local doctors and the experts than there was over DR patients. The first expert passed the ENT management in 34 cases out of 49 requiring further management. The second passed 31 cases out of 48 (one was rated a 'don't know'). The average MPE rate is 67%, and this is substantially higher than the figure of 32% for doctors seeing DR patients. In fact, there are a number of reasons for believing that, on the whole, the ENT safety-checks on DR patients were done to a less stringent standard than usual, and this point is discussed later.

10.8.11 *Management of Potentially serious Conditions in TR Patients.* On the first expert's figures ENT doctors appropriately managed 7 out of 17 potentially serious TR cases; and on the second expert's figures it was 9 out of 22. Both of these produce an MPE rate of 41%. This is somewhat higher than the average of 26% for doctors seeing DRs.

10.8.12 The MPE rates for both technicians and doctors – particularly for the latter – appear rather low. However, closer investigation reveals that much of the discrepancy from the 'Gold Standard' set by the specialists and experts appears to be due to differences of opinion over the way that certain conditions should be managed, rather than to outright mistakes. This point is considered in detail in the 'Summary and discussion' section following the presentation of results.

10.9 Results – comparison of TR and DR systems
(table 10.7)

10.9.1 Although it was felt to be inappropriate to compare technicians and doctors with regard to management performance, it is perfectly valid to directly compare the DR and TR *systems* of provision. The aim here is to compare the proportions of patients under each system who go through with significant pathology remaining undetected. For the TR system this is the same as the proportion missed by doctors. With regard to DR however, the total for the *system* is a combination of failures by technicians and failures by doctors. Specifically, the total failures consist of those cases where the technician failed to cross-refer a patient with pathology *plus* those cases where the technician did cross but the doctor missed the pathology. These are cases which in a normal DR system would go through the system with undetected conditions.

10.9.2 *Management of Patients.* On the basis of the first expert's assessments, out of 21 DR patients (excluding incomplete cases) needing further

Table 10.7

Comparison of TR and DR systems

Management of pathology when present – all cases needing further management

		No. of passes	No. needing management	Pass rate
DR SYSTEM	Expert 1	5	21	24%
	Expert 2	8	20	40%
TR SYSTEM	Expert 1	34	49	69%
	Expert 2	31	48	65%

Management of pathology when present – potentially serious cases only

		No. of passes	No. serious cases	Pass rate
DR SYSTEM	Expert 1	1	7	14%
	Expert 2	4	12	33%
TR SYSTEM	Expert 1	7	17	41%
	Expert 2	9	22	41%

Overall rates of failures of management

		No. of fails	Total cases	Failure rate
DR SYSTEM	Expert 1	16	234	6.8%
	Expert 2	12	233	5.2%
TR SYSTEM	Expert 1	15	211	7.1%
	Expert 2	17	210	8.1%

Overall rates of potentially serious failures of management

		Pot. serious fails	Total cases	Failure rate
DR SYSTEM	Expert 1	6	234	2.6%
	Expert 2	8	233	3.4%
TR SYSTEM	Expert 1	10	211	4.7%
	Expert 2	13	210	6.2%

Note: cases with a missing technician or doctor pro-forma (or a 'don't know' rating) have been excluded.

management just 5 (24%) received it. This compares to 34 out of 49 appropriately managed under TR (69%). The corresponding figures for the second expert were 8 out of 20 under DR (40%) and 31 out of 48 under TR (65%). These figures yield average MPE rates of 32% for DR patients, compared to 67% for TR patients. The difference between systems is highly significant on the first experts figures (chi-square with Yates correction = 10.6, $p<0.01$), but not significant on those of the second (chi-square with Yates correction = 2.56, $p>0.05$, also not significant as a raw chi-square).

10.9.3 Whereas the above suggests that a higher proportion of DR patients who need further management may not receive it, when considered in the context of all patients coming through the systems the difference disappears completely: the average rate of management success over all DR patients was 94%, and over all TR patients it was 92.4%. The reason why the difference in favour of TR disappears is because many more of these patients needed management in the first place. In all, there were 11 DR cases that both experts regarded as management failures compared to 10 TR cases.

10.9.4 Chi-squared tests on the overall rates were not significant for either expert.

10.9.5 *Management of Potentially Serious Conditions.* On the first expert's assessments, just 1 out of a total of 7 DR patients with potentially serious conditions received appropriate management. It is worth noting that 4 of the 6 management failures were in fact cross-referred by technicians, but were considered by the ENT doctor to require no action other than hearing aid fitting.

10.9.6 The MPE rate of 1 out of 7 for DR (14%) compares with a rate of 7 out of 17 for TR (41%). The corresponding results for the second expert were 4 out of 12 potentially serious cases acceptably managed under DR (33%) as against 9 out of 22 under TR (41%). These results suggest an average MPE rate with regard to the *management of potentially serious conditions when present* of 24% for the DR system against 41% for the TR system. However, on chi-square tests the difference is not statistically significant for either expert, and it must be emphasised that the samples are very small.

10.9.7 Rates of potentially serious failures across all patients seen for the two systems were 2.6% for DR against 4.7% for TR according to the first expert, and 3.4% against 6.2% according to the second. These yield an average of 3.0% for DR and 5.5% for TR. That is, on the basis of the expert assessments, around 1 in every 33 DR patients goes through the system with a potentially serious condition remaining unmanaged compared to 1 in 18 TR patients.

10.9.8 There were 5 DR cases considered by both experts to be potentially serious failures, compared to 6 TR cases.

10.10 Results – comparison of a mix of DR and TR systems with TR alone

10.10.1 As a rule, Hearing Aid Centres operate a combination of DR and TR systems, with some patients coming through the former and some through the latter. It is appropriate therefore to ask what numbers of management failures can be expected when a *combination of the two systems* is operating compared to if TR were operating alone. This is perhaps the most appropriate way to assess the increased risk of introducing Direct Referral, as this is the situation usually found in practice. For simplicity, the analysis here is restricted solely to the management of potentially serious conditions.

10.10.2 To address this question, a somewhat more sophisticated approach was needed than the straightforward counts of management passes and fails that have been presented up to now. This involved one or two rather complex estimations, and to avoid cluttering up the text these are presented in appendix I.IV.

10.10.3 The analysis makes the assumption that under a normal DR system ENT doctors will apply the same standards of examination to cross-referred DR patients as they do to TR patients. However, there is evidence (discussed later) that the special circumstances of the pilot schemes (specifically, the requirement that *all* DR patients be seen by ENT) resulted in the safety-checks being done to a lower standard than normal ENT examinations. In view of this, calculations throughout have been based on the observed ENT MPE rate with the TR sample, which we consider to more representative of what would happen under a 'normal' DR system.

10.10.4 On the first expert's findings technicians correctly cross-refer 50% of DR patients with potentially serious conditions, and ENT doctors can be expected to appropriately manage 41% of these (based on their performance with TR patients). Therefore, on the basis of the findings of this expert, the proportion of patients with potentially serious conditions who can be expected to be picked up under the DR system is 0.5*0.41 = 21% (this compares to 41% under the TR system).

10.10.5 It is also estimated (on this experts findings, see appendix I.IV) that in the latter part of the project period around 77% of all patients with potentially serious pathology were coming through TR, and the remaining 23% through DR. On this basis, relative to a MPE rate under TR of 41%, the proportion of potentially serious conditions expected to be picked up under *the mix of both systems* is 0.21*0.23 + 0.41*0.77 = 36%. This suggests a difference between the mixed DR/TR system and TR alone of 5% in favour of the latter. That is, the introduction of DR increases the risk to patients (i.e. the chance of going through the provision process with a potentially serious condition remaining undetected) by 5%. It is of interest to note that this figure of 5% increased risk is relatively unaffected by the estimated rates of management failure by local doctors. For example, if the 'true' rate of ENT management failure was, say, 30% instead of the estimated 59%, then the level of increased risk becomes 8% instead of 5%.

10.10.6 Approximate 95% confidence limits on the estimate of a 5% difference have been computed treating both technician and doctor success rates as variables (appendix I.IV). These suggest that the true value lies within the range of 1% to 9%.

10.10.7 Calculations based on the second expert's findings produce a very similar result. Using his figures it is estimated that 25% of all potentially serious cases go through DR, technicians successfully detect 57% of these, and doctors appropriately manage 41%. On this basis, it is calculated that 23% of potentially serious cases coming through DR will be properly managed; and that under the combination of DR and TR systems the MPE rate will be 37%, in comparison with 41% under TR alone. These results are almost identical to those for the first expert. An approximate 95% confidence interval on the difference in rates indicates its true value to lie between 1% and 8% in favour of TR alone.

10.10.8 It needs to be noted that the above findings are based on the assumption that the proportion of potentially serious cases coming through DR is around the estimated values of 23% to 25%. A lower proportion than this would result in the MPE rates being even closer; but a higher proportion enhances the advantage of TR operating on its own. Theoretically, however, the percentage of potentially serious conditions being referred via DR is highly unlikely to exceed 50% (which would imply that GPs have zero success in identifying pathology). Under this assumption, the expected MPE rates are 31% – 32% for DR/TR mixed as against 41% for TR alone.

10.10.9 These results have been used to derive failure rates over all patients seen. On the first expert's assessments, under the DR/TR mix some 4.3% of all patients would be potentially serious failures, as against 4.0% if all patients came through TR. The corresponding rates for the second expert are 5.9% compared to 5.6%. The difference in this respect between a mixed service and TR alone therefore appears very small indeed, just 0.3%. This amounts to no more than one extra potentially serious failure in every 300 patients. The upper 95% confidence limit on this figure is about 1 in every 150 patients.

10.10.10 Some confirmation of this result comes from the comparison of technicians with local ENT doctors over the pilot projects as a whole (chapter 9). The data from that exercise (a total sample of over 2,300 patients) allowed us to estimate that the rate of additional potentially serious failures under the combination of DR and TR – compared to if all patients had come through TR – was about 1 in every 430 patients seen (section 9.8). This figure is not too different from the present estimate of 1 in 300. A rate of 1 in 430 is equivalent to an increased risk of potentially serious pathology being missed in the order of about 3.5%. Given, however, the evidence that some of the ENT safety-checks on DR patients during the pilots were less stringent than a normal ENT examination, this figure is likely to slightly underestimate the true value.

10.11 Summary and discussion

10.11.1 The comparative safety of the Direct Referral procedure has been studied in three different ways: by examining the performance of technicians and of ENT doctors; by comparing rates of management failure under DR with those under TR; and by evaluating the increased risk of a mixed DR/TR service over TR operating on its own.

10.11.2 The technicians and ENT doctors who examined patients have been looked at in terms of three measures of performance: diagnosis, management, and management of potentially serious conditions. Technicians were judged by the experts to have appropriately managed 61% of all DR cases needing further management, and to have correctly cross-referred 54% of the potentially serious cases. On the same sample of DR patients (bar incomplete cases), doctors managed 32% of all conditions, and 26% of potentially serious conditions, to the satisfaction of the experts. There was less discrepancy between the experts and local doctors with regard to TR patients: here, 67% of all conditions, and 41% of potentially serious conditions, were judged to have been satisfactorily managed.

10.11.3 The results for ENT doctors suggest a substantial difference between themselves and the expert assessors. Several factors may be contributing to this, other than actual 'mistakes' by local doctors. One factor concerns the wide variety of opinion that exists between ENT doctors over the management of individual cases. The opinion of the expert assessors has been taken as the 'Gold Standard' against which the performance of local doctors has been evaluated; however, a considerable difference was found between the experts themselves. For example, over the DR and TR samples combined expert 1 identified 16 potentially serious failures of management by local doctors, but expert 2 considered 5 of these to be management passes: that is, if expert 1 was 'right' then expert 2 was 'wrong' in 31% of cases. Another factor to consider is that – unlike the local doctors – the experts were not making their decisions in the circumstances of a busy ENT clinic with both time and resource constraints to consider: if they had been some of their decisions, particularly with borderline cases, may have been different. A third consideration is that the experts did not see the patients face-to-face (although the specialists – who earmarked them as needing further management – did), and so were not able to take other aspects of the patient's general health or personality into account in their decisions.

10.11.4 It is not likely that the above factors can account for all the differences between the experts and local doctors, however. Rather, the major factor operating here appears to be a *difference over the management of asymmetrical hearing loss.* 70% of the cases rated as potentially serious ENT failures involved asymmetrical loss, which can indicate a possible acoustic neuroma. All of these cases the experts (as well as the specialists) had felt should be investigated, but in the main the local doctors had been content to discharge these patients. In our discussions with ENT doctors it became clear that there exists a division of opinion over the management of such cases. Many doctors take the view that, with elderly patients, even if one were to investigate and identify a tumour, the stress of an operation may well do more harm than just leaving it alone, and therefore often even the investigation is not worth doing. Other doctors believe that in many such cases investigation and treatment is worthwhile. It was clear that the experts and external specialists took the latter position, while most – but not all – of the local doctors apparently took the former.

10.11.5 In this context, it is instructive to consider the DR cases that technicians failed to cross. More than half of the potentially serious fails by technicians involved asymmetrical loss (as did 9 out of the 15 potentially serious fails across all DR patients seen during the pilots – see section 9.9). These asymmetries in fact all fail the TTSA guidelines. The likely reason why these cases were not cross-referred is that technicians tend to work to what they perceive to be the criteria of their own ENT doctors. Thus if a large proportion of the patients with asymmetrical losses they cross-refer are sent straight back with no action taken, technicians may tend to stop making such cross-referrals. This observation ties in with the point made previously about differing ENT attitudes to the management of such cases: for example, we have heard technicians expressing the same opinion as many doctors that asymmetrical losses in elderly patients are not worth investigating. This highlights the fact that it may be difficult to change technician practice unless ENT practice also changes. Also, it suggests that many of the technician 'errors' were a consequence of the local philosophy of management differing from that of the specialists and experts, and not outright mistakes.

10.11.6 The issue of what the correct management in such cases should be is well beyond the scope of the present study, but would certainly appear to be a matter that the ENT community needs to address, given the findings of this research.

10.11.7 We turn now to the comparison of DR and TR as *systems* of provision. Failure rates for Direct Referral as a system are necessarily higher than for technicians alone. This is because even if a technician correctly detects a significant abnormality and cross-refers, there is a chance that the examining ENT doctor will fail to correctly manage the condition. Even so, in terms of numbers of failures out of all patients seen, the rates for DR were lower than for TR whether one looks at all management failures or only potentially serious failures, but not significantly so. The overall indication from the expert assessments was that under the DR system about 3% of patients had a potentially serious condition that was not managed, compared to 5.5% of TR patients.

10.11.8 In considering this finding however, it is important to recall that the incidence of patients with potentially serious conditions was much lower in the DR sample to begin with. When the rates of detection of pathology *when present* were compared the TR system came out better, with around 41% of potentially serious cases being detected compared to 24% under DR. Although both figures look small, it must be emphasised that they are calculated relative to the opinions of the two experts, and for reasons discussed previously may well be unduly low. Although the difference was not significant, the samples involved were very small.

10.11.9 As a rule, Hearing Aid Centres which operate DR do so in parallel with the Traditional Referral system. It was estimated that during the latter phase of the pilots around one-quarter of all potentially serious cases were coming through the DR systems. On this basis, it has been calculated that relative to a rate of detection of potentially serious conditions under TR by itself of 41%, the mix of DR and TR systems would detect about 36%. That is, about 5% of all patients with potentially serious conditions who would be picked up under TR will be missed under the combination of DR and TR systems. Confidence limits on this figure (treating both rates as variables) indicate that the true value is unlikely to exceed 9%. Also, these results are relatively unaffected by the issue of the 'accuracy' of the ENT 'failure' rates. Expressed in terms of a rate of potentially serious management failures over all patients seen, the increased risk from introducing DR appears very low indeed, amounting to no more than around 1 additional potentially serious failure in every 300 patients.

10.11.10 With regard to the preceding, an important theoretical point needs to be made. The calculations involved in comparing a DR/TR mix with TR alone have been based on the assumption that ENT doctors apply *the same standards whether seeing TR or DR patients*. However, there are good reasons for believing that during the pilots many doctors applied *lower* standards to DR patients, but that in a 'normal' DR system they would probably apply *higher* standards.

10.11.11 With regard to the pilot schemes, it was clear that at many Centres ENT doctors were not that interested in doing the safety-checks. There were large numbers to do (because all DR patients were checked), and the vast majority were straightforward, which made the exercise rather boring. Also, the fact that these were Direct Referrals must have lowered expectations of finding anything clinically significant. It is shown in a later chapter that many doctors spent considerably less time on the checks than they would with a TR patient.

10.11.12 Another factor was that Centres tended not to make much distinction between crossed and uncrossed patients because all had to be seen by a doctor anyway, and furthermore, technicians were asked not to reveal the details of the examinations they had done to the safety-check doctors, so as to avoid influencing the latter.

10.11.13 Under a 'normal' DR system only the cross-referred patients would be seen in ENT. Because the technician had made a special point of cross-referring, the doctor would be alerted to the fact that there may well be something significant present. Also, the doctor would have access to the details of the technician's findings and know the specific reason for cross-referral. Under these conditions, doctors might well make less errors than during the pilot schemes. Furthermore, these factors may well make them take a harder look at these cross-referrals than they do at TR patients, if they have a higher expectation of finding something significant.

10.11.14 The question remains as to whether these considerations would be sufficient to overcome the estimated disadvantage of the DR/TR mix compared to TR alone. On the evidence of present data ENT doctors would need to be nearly *twice* as successful in detecting potentially serious pathology in cross-referred DR patients as they are in TRs for the differential to be *completely eliminated* (this is because technicians crossed only just over half of the potentially serious cases). It seems unlikely that such a large change would occur, and therefore the issue is one of whether the increased level of risk under a DR/TR mix – estimated to be between 1% and 9% for patients with potentially serious conditions – is acceptable or not.

10.11.15 In considering this question, there are a number of factors which should be taken into account. Firstly, we are talking here of *potentially* serious failures – a proportion of which might well, in the event, prove to be not serious at all. Secondly, the missed cases are not necessarily 'lost for ever', as any ear disease present may possibly be picked up at subsequent visits to their GP. Thirdly, and perhaps most crucially, the level of increased risk involved is probably much smaller than the degree of variation that already exists between different ENT doctors. That is, it is less than the potential risk increase due to being seen by one ENT doctor rather than another. For example, it was observed earlier (10.11.3) that 31% of cases regarded as potentially serious failures of management by expert 1 were considered management passes by expert 2. This suggests - under the assumption that expert 1 is correct – a 31% increased risk of potentially serious disease being missed for expert 2.

10.11.16 Also to be considered is the fact that DR removes substantial numbers of straightforward hearing aid patients from ENT clinic queues. This should lead to other ENT patients with possibly serious conditions being seen and treated at an earlier date than they otherwise would have, and this factor off-sets the risk increase to some degree.

10.11.17 A final factor is the observation that at many Centres the current practice is for TR patients referred for hearing aids to be selected out and seen by junior ENT doctors. A DR scheme operated by highly experienced technicians in which all cross-referrals are seen by senior ENT staff could in fact prove to be more safe than this arrangement.

10.11.18 There is also the possibility of taking practical steps to minimise the level of increased risk. One step would be to ensure that technicians follow the guidelines for cross-referral carefully. It has been mentioned that a high proportion of the technician failures involved asymmetrical loss, and it should not be too difficult to reduce this by setting clear and precise criteria and enforcing strict adherence to them. Another step would be to make certain that all patients cross-referred by technicians are seen only by doctors with a high degree of experience. Also, the general issue of how best to manage elderly patients exhibiting asymmetrical loss needs to be addressed by the ENT community. Lastly, everything possible should be done to encourage GPs to do a better job of detecting disease themselves so that they only refer appropriate patients.

10.12 Experimental factors

10.12.1 There are a number of factors to do with the conditions of the experiment which require some discussion. This is because they have a bearing upon the validity of the findings.

10.12.2 The first consideration is whether experimental conditions were the same for technicians and ENT doctors. On the whole, it is probable that technicians were more conscious than doctors of the fact that the results of their patient examinations were going to be evaluated by external assessors. The Hearing Aid Centres made the arrangements for the external specialist visits, and while ENT departments were certainly aware that the trials were being undertaken, many doctors may have only been vaguely aware of the specific dates involved or the object of the exercise. It may be, therefore, that knowing when the specialists were coming, some technicians 'tried harder' in the period preceding the visits, while perhaps doctors did not. This would tend to enhance the difference between the two groups.

10.12.3 A second factor is that the expert assessors did not see the patients' conditions for themselves, but based their assessments upon the recorded findings of the external specialists, and copies of audiograms, ENT notes, and completed examination pro-formas. This factor may account for some of the discrepancy between their conclusions and the management decisions of technicians and local doctors, and also for some of the discrepancy between the experts themselves. However, given that this factor affects the results for both the DR and TR samples, it does not alter the findings regarding the *comparative* safety of the two systems. For example, computations based on only those cases considered potentially serious by *both* experts yield an almost identical result as previous, of around 1 extra potentially serious management failure in every 300 patients as a result of introducing DR.

10.12.4 The information available to the expert assessors did differ between the DR and TR samples, however, in that for TR patients assessment of the local doctor's management was made on the basis of copies of the ENT examination notes, whereas for DR patients it was based on the pro-formas they completed. This raises the question of how compatible the different sources of information were.

10.12.5 Regarding the ENT notes, in the great majority of cases copies of the letter sent by the examining doctor to the referring GP regarding the results of the ENT examination were also available, and these were normally quite specific about the major findings and management decisions. With the pro-formas on the other hand, doctors ticked boxes indicating the findings and decisions. However, our impression was that a number of doctors were not as thorough in this as they could have been, and in some cases may have made findings or management decisions they did not record. However, if it is true that important information was missing for more DR than TR patients, this would lead the experts to incorrectly fail more DR than TR cases (e.g. if an ENT doctor intended to do further investigation but did not indicate this on the pro-forma, the expert would assume that he had discharged the patient). Therefore, this factor mainly operates against DR, and so if anything the actual comparative safety of the system is better than the present results indicate.

10.12.6 Another factor relates to both TR and DR samples more or less equally. Neither the ENT notes nor the pro-formas contained details of conversations between doctors and patients. Thus it may be that in some cases management options were discussed with the patient (e.g. whether to operate or not), but only the decision was recorded (e.g. no management other than an aid). This could have produced a number of 'false' management failures (e.g the expert may have felt that an operation should be offered, and presumed that one was not). The experts were asked to give a rating of 'don't know' in cases where they could not decide if the case was managed correctly, but this rating was rarely used.

10.12.7 Given that the above is a possibility, it may be that rates of failure for both the TR and DR systems were in actuality lower than the results of the experiment suggest.

10.12.8 A final consideration is one that has been mentioned previously in the discussion section. This is the fact that there is good evidence to believe that the doctors seeing cross-referrals were in many cases not as thorough as they would be if the DR system were operating in normal circumstances. This would imply that in a normal situation the number of management failures under DR would be less than in the experiment.

10.12.9 In summary, only one of the experimental factors discussed above could be expected to have produced a bias in favour of the DR system (that technicians might have taken extra care knowing that their work was being evaluated). In contrast, however, there are a number of other factors which, if anything, operate in the opposite direction, suggesting that the results most likely underestimate the comparative safety of DR.

10.13 Grades of technicians and doctors committing potentially serious management failures

10.13.1 *Doctors*. All grades of ENT doctors are represented amongst the potentially serious failures (with the exception of house officers, but no patients in the samples were seen by this grade). Combining the TR and DR samples for simplicity, on the ratings of the first expert 2 potentially serious failures were by consultants, 3 by senior registrars, 3 by registrars, 2 by SHOs, and 3 by clinical assistants. The second expert found 6 by consultants, 6 by registrars, 1 by an SHO, and 5 by clinical assistants. (There were 3 other potentially serious failures where the doctor's grade was not known).

10.13.2 With regard to potentially serious failures by technicians, the first Expert found 2 by MTO5s and 3 by MTO4s. The second found 2 by MTO5s, 2 by MTO4s, and 2 by MTO3s. As with doctors, the failures are spread across the range of technician grades.

10.13.3 No potentially serious management failures by private dispensers were identified. 35 of the DR patients examined by the external specialists had originally been seen by a private dispenser (15% of the total). However, only one was considered by them to require anything more than a hearing aid, and so this was the only one assessed by the independent experts. Both experts failed the dispenser on both diagnosis and management, but one regarded the patients condition as not serious, and the other as moderately serious.

10.14 Comment by external specialists

10.14.1 The two external specialists were invited to make a personal comment on the medical visits they had done, on the understanding that these would appear in the report unedited. Mr Smith provided a page of comments, which is presented in Appendix I.VI.

11   Other Aspects of Quality Assurance

11.1 Queuing times
(tables 11.1 and 11.2)

11.1.1 TR and DR patients who were interviewed were asked how long they had queued in the waiting room prior to being seen at each appointment. Table 11.1 compares the queuing times of TR patients waiting for their examination by an ENT doctor with those of DR patients waiting to be examined by a technician. Patients who were seen late because they arrived late for the appointment have been excluded. Percentages are given for patients who were seen within 10 minutes, which can be regarded as a short wait, and those who queued 30 minutes or more, which is a fairly long wait. Patients answered this question on a retrospective basis, and the original appointments were on a great variety of different dates. Therefore the figures should be fairly representative, and are not simply reflections of the service on a particular day or few days.

Table 11.1

Queuing times at examination appointment (figures in percentages)

| | Seen within 10 minutes | | Queued 30 mins or more | | Sample size | |
	TR	DR	TR	DR	TR	DR
Orange	82%	no data	9%	no data	11	nd
Red	69	88	6	0	16	16
Yellow	82	81	0	5	17	21
Green	35	62	55	15	20	13
Blue(NH)	no data	82	no data	6	nd	17
Blue(PD)	not applicable	89	not applicable	11	na	9
White	71	94	17	0	17	18
Black	no data	65	no data	20	nd	20
Grey	31	77	19	23	16	13
Brown	60	100	20	0	15	18
Silver	67	100	28	0	21	20
Gold	37	100	63	0	19	18
Bronze	44	100	50	0	16	21
Overall*	55%	91%	30%	4%	157	158

*Overall figures are based on Centres with TR and DR data only.

11.1.2 With regards to TR patients there is a great deal of variation between Centres, with the percentage seen within 10 minutes varying from just 31% at Grey up to 82% at Orange and Yellow. In terms of patients queuing for half an hour or more, the poorest services were Gold (63%), Green (55%), and Bronze (50%).

Table 11.2
Queuing times at fitting
appointment (figures in
percentages)

	Seen within 10 minutes		Queued 30 mins or more		Sample size	
	TR	DR	TR	DR	TR	DR
Orange	91%	no data	0%	no data	11	nd
Red	89	100	0	0	18	14
Yellow	72	80	6	10	18	20
Green	85	64	5	0	20	11
Blue(NH)	no data	94	no data	0	nd	17
Blue(PD)	not applicable	100	not applicable	0	na	10
White	89	88	0	0	18	17
Black	no data	100	no data	0	nd	20
Grey	63	82	21	6	19	17
Brown	89	95	0	0	18	20
Silver	86	100	9	0	22	21
Gold	100	100	0	0	19	18
Bronze	90	86	0	0	19	21
Overall*	85%	89%	5%	2%	171	159

*Overall figures are based on Centres with TR and DR data only.

11.1.3 DR patients generally experienced shorter queuing times. The poorest service was at Green, where just 62% were seen within 10 minutes. In contrast, at four Centres (Silver, Brown, Gold, and Bronze) 100% of DR patients were seen within this time. At six Centres no patients queued for half an hour, and the worst figure anywhere was 23%, at Grey. Overall, 91% of DR patients were seen within 10 minutes compared to 55% of TR patients, and 4% queued for 30 minutes or more compared to 30% of TRs.

11.1.4 Table 11.2 compares the queuing times at the appointment for hearing aid fitting for TR and DR patients. The vast majority of patients were interviewed at the time of fitting, and so for most Centres the figures represent the service on only a few particular days (when interviewing took place). Also, it is possible that technicians 'tried harder' on those days given the presence of the interviewers. On the other hand, however, the actual times reported by patients are likely to be more accurate because the interviewing took place within an hour of queuing.

11.1.5 The results for the two groups are very similar, with (overall) 85% of TRs queuing 10 minutes or less, and 89% of DRs. These figures are also very close to the 91% figure for queuing times of DR patients at the examination appointment. The closeness of all three sets of results suggests that the figures are a fairly reliable and accurate measure of the time patients spend waiting to be seen by a technician.

11.2 Number of appointments to point of fitting
(table 11.3)

11.2.1 The analysis here covers all appointments after GP referral to do with provision of the aid. Follow-up appointments after fitting are not included. Data collection on patients did not extend beyond the appointment for fitting, and although the great majority of Centres arranged follow-ups, it was clear that a substantial, but unknown, proportion of patients did not attend these.

Table 11.3

Number of appointments up to point of fitting

	Traditional referral 2	3+	DR excluding cross-referral 2	3+	DR including cross-referral 2	3+	Sample size TR	DR
Orange	75%	25%	— no data —				20	nd
Red	29	71	47	53	not known		17	17
Yellow	84	6	95	5	62	38	19	21
Green	94	6	100	0	71	29	17	14
Blue(NH)	94	6	18	82	12	88	17	17
Blue(PD)	not applicable		40	60	40	60	na	10
White	81	19	35	65	29	71	16	17
Black	no data		59	41	45	55	nd	22
Grey	12	88	79	21	74	26	17	19
Brown	53	47	84	16	79	21	15	19
Silver	94	6	76	24	76	24	18	21
Gold	88	12	89	11	67	33	16	18
Bronze	88	12	59	41	50	50	16	22
Overall*	76%	24%	71%	29%	58%	42%	152	168

*Overall figures are based on Centres with TR and DR data only.

11.2.2 The analysis is based upon information from the TR and DR patients who were interviewed, as this data yielded the fullest information about appointments attended. Only patients who were referred by GPs have been included in the analysis (a small number referred by other hospital departments were excluded).

11.2.3 The analysis covers all appointments at the hospital, both those related to the usual procedures (ear examination, audio testing, ear impressions, fitting, and cross-referral ENT examination (DRs only)); and the less common ones (a separate appointment for dewaxing, additional testing, additional ear impressions etc). In addition to the above, also included are any visits to the GP for wax removal subsequent to referral. A number of Centres requested DR patients to go back to their GP before attending the hospital to have any wax removed, and this is an additional GP appointment not normally experienced by TR patients. At some Centres high proportions of DR patients had this extra appointment: in several cases it was over 50%, and the highest was 82%, at Blue(NH). Also, a few other DR patients found to have significant wax upon attending the Centre were sent back to their GP for dewaxing.

11.2.4 Several of the procedures can be carried out in one visit. The most common approach is for the ENT examination (or technician examination for DRs), audio testing and ear impressions to be undertaken at the first appointment, and the fitting at a second appointment. The great majority of TR patients are seen to in just two visits. Most DR patients are also served in two visits. The principal exceptions to this are those cross-referred to ENT (which often involves an extra appointment), and those asked to return to their GP for dewaxing.

11.2.5 A difficulty arose with the data in that in most cases it was not known whether a DR patient had been cross-referred or not. To overcome this, a proportion of DR interviewees at each Centre were treated 'as if' they had been cross-referred. The proportions were equal to the overall percentages crossed at each Centre, and random numbers were used to select the cases treated in this way. It needs to be noted that the management of cross-referrals changed after the end of the project period such that virtually all cross-referrals are now seen in ENT as a separate appointment, and not on the same day as one of the other appointments. It was felt that the analysis of appointments should reflect this situation , rather than the more artificial one that existed during the pilot period. Therefore, all instances of cross-referral have been treated as involving a separate appointment for the patient. The exception to this is Gold, where the ENT consultant decides on the basis of the technician's report whether or not to recall a patient. Only the proportion actually called in for examination are counted as having an extra appointment.

11.2.6 Amongst the patients interviewed, only a very small percentage of either group required more than three appointments: just 4.2% of all TRs, and a somewhat higher proportion, 7%, of all DRs. Only two patients (1 TR and 1 DR out of a total of 406) had 5 appointments, and just 1 DR patient needed 6 (which included two returns to the GP for dewax). Consequently, for simplicity the results have been collapsed to just two categories: two appointments, and three or more.

11.2.7 Regarding TR patients, at most Centres only a small percentage required more than 2 appointments; at seven places it was less than 20%. However, there were two places where the proportion was very high. At Grey it was 88%; but this Centre experienced severe cuts in technician staff shortly before the project start, and had to abandon technician support for community ENT clinics. At Red it was 71%, and this was almost entirely due to TR patients being asked to return to their GP for dewax before attending (unusual for a TR service). Although figures are not available for Black, it is known that at this Centre nearly all TR patients had at least three appointments, as a result of the service here being split across two sites.

11.2.8 The second set of figures in table 11.3 gives percentages for the DR cases excluding any cross-referral appointments. The results are far more variable than for TRs. However, in those cases where the numbers having three or more appointments were substantial (most notably Blue(NH) 82%; White 65%; Red 53%; and Black and Bronze 41%), nearly all of this was due to returns to the GP for wax removal.

11.2.9 The table also gives percentages for DR patients taking into account appointments for cross-referral. When these are included, at several Centres the proportion of DRs being served in two appointments is considerably lower than the corresponding proportion for TR patients. The most dramatic cases are Blue(NH) where it is just 12% compared to 94%, and White (29% as against 81%). In all, at seven Centres more TRs than DRs were seen in 2 appointments, and there are just two where the opposite prevailed. Over-all, 76% of TR patients were served in 2 appointments, as against 58% of DR patients.

11.3 Time spent by patients on travelling and appointments
(table 11.4)

11.3.1 At the interviews, both TR and DR patients were asked a number of questions concerning the amount of time they had spent on appointments, both travelling and at the appointment.

Table 11.4
Time spent by patients on travelling and appointments

	Traditional Referral	Straightforward Direct Referral	Direct Referral plus cross-referral	All DR patients (see A)
Orange	3hrs 56mins	———————— no data ————————		
Red	4hrs 36mins	4hrs 40mins	6hrs 27mins	not known
Yellow	3hrs 40mins	2hrs 39mins	4hrs 9mins	3hrs 13mins
Green	3hrs 51mins	2hrs 49mins	4hrs 48mins	3hrs 23mins
Blue(NH)	3hrs 55mins	4hrs 17mins	5hrs 30mins	4hrs 30mins
Blue(PD)	not applicable	3hrs 0mins	4hr 13mins	3hrs 8mins
White	4hrs 1mins	3hrs 17mins	4hrs 47mins	3hrs 38mins
Black	no data	4hrs 3mins	5hrs 53mins	4hrs 23mins
Grey	5hrs 51mins	2hrs 39mins	4hrs 10mins	2hrs 49mins
Brown	4hrs 38mins	1hr 55mins	3hrs 23mins	2hrs 0mins
Silver	3hrs 26mins	3hrs 22mins	4hrs 46mins	3hrs 30mins
Gold	3hrs 25mins	2hrs 58mins	5hrs 4min	3hrs 26mins
Bronze	3hrs 53mins	2hrs 57mins	4hrs 49mins	3hrs 7mins
Mean*	4hrs 4mins	2hrs 59mins	4hrs 36mins	3hrs 17mins

*Mean based on Centres with both TR and DR data only.
A) Average time for all DR patients, including appointments for cross-referral and returns to GP for dewax.
NOTE ON SAMPLE SIZES: Figures are sums across various appointments, with varying sample sizes. For TR, samples varied between 15 and 22; for DR between 12 and 22.

11.3.2 For both groups of patients, the analysis covers the same appointments as were considered in the previous section. That is: all appointments at the hospital/Centre related to provision (up to the point of fitting), plus any appointments at the GP for dewaxing subsequent to referral. The initial visit to the GP is not included.

11.3.3 The results should be regarded as very approximate. They are based principally upon recollections and estimates made by patients. In addition, the sample sizes involved are quite small: no more than 20 TR or DR patients at any Centre.

11.3.4 The table contains four columns. The first is times spent by TR patients. These are derived from the information given by interviewed TR patients. The second column is times for DR without any cross-referral. These are based on DR patient interviews; note that some of the patients may actually have been cross-referred, but the time spent on the cross-referral has been excluded.

11.3.5 Computation of the times in the third column – for DR plus cross-referral – was more complicated. There was very little detail from the patients themselves about cross-referral appointments: only a few were cross-referred, and many of these had not been seen in ENT yet. Therefore, for each Centre an average time spent on a cross-referral ENT appointment was estimated using the information from TR patients about their ENT appointments.

11.3.6 To do this, the average time spent by each TR patient at the Centre on the first appointment was taken, and from this was subtracted average times (at that Centre) for audio testing and ear impressions (unless done at a different appointment, see table 15.6 for these times) to give an estimate of the time spent on the ENT examination alone. All cross-referrals were treated as involving a separate appointment so as to duplicate 'normal' DR practice (see paragraph 11.2.5), and therefore travelling time was added. The resulting figure was then added to the times for straightforward DR patients to give an estimate for DR plus cross-referral.

11.3.7 Column four in the table gives overall means for all DR patients. That is, both straightforward and cross-referred patients, in the proportions found in the projects.

11.3.8 *TR Patients*. The times spent by TR patients vary between 3hrs 25mins and 5hrs 51mins. Not surprisingly, the two Centres with the highest times – Grey and Brown – were those where substantial numbers of TR patients had three appointments rather than the more usual two.

11.3.9 *Straightforward DR Patients*. The times for straightforward DR provision (i.e. no cross-referral) range between 1hr 55mins and 4hrs 40mins. They are lower than for TR at all Centres excepting Red and Blue(NH). At most Centres, the reduction is due mainly to the fact that DR patients did not experience the long queuing times to see the ENT doctor that many in the TR group endured. Overall (Centres with full data only), the mean time spent by straightforward DR patients was 2hrs 59mins, compared to 4hrs 4mins for TR patients.

11.3.10 There are very large time reductions at Grey and Brown (down by 3hrs 12mins and 2hrs 43mins, respectively). Both of these reductions are due principally to DR patients being seen by technicians at local community clinics in two appointments, whereas most TR patients were seen locally by an ENT doctor but then had a further two appointments at the main site Hearing Aid Centre. In both cases at least half the time saving was due to reduced patient travelling times.

11.3.11 *Cross-referred DR patients*. Although at most Centres straightforward DR patients spend less time on appointments than their TR colleagues, when an extra cross-referral appointment at ENT is included the times for DR are generally higher than for TR. This is true at every Centre except Grey and Brown (for reasons given previously). The extra time spent on the cross-referral varies between 1hr 13mins and 2hrs 6mins. Most of the larger increments are due to queuing times at the ENT department.

11.3.12 *All DR Patients.* When both straightforward and cross-referred DRs are taken together, in the proportions found in the pilots, the average times spent by each patient range between a low of 2hrs and a high of 4hrs 30mins. The times are lower than those for TR patients at six Centres, much the same at two, and higher at just one. The largest time saving is over 2 hours. Overall (comparable Centres only) the average time spent on appointments by a TR patient was 4hrs 4mins, and for a DR patient it was 3hrs 17mins.

11.4 Patient satisfaction with service

11.4.1 Assessing patient satisfaction with this population presented some special problems. Nearly all of the patients were elderly – a substantial proportion very elderly – and by definition they were hard of hearing. Consequently there were communication problems with quite a proportion, plus additional difficulties with those whose memories or health was poor. Fortunately, many of the more severely handicapped patients attended with friends or relatives, who acted as 'interpreters' or answered on the patient's behalf.

11.4.2 During the initial interviewing sessions, an attempt was made to use Lickert-type satisfaction rating scales. The problems alluded to above caused great difficulties in getting patients to understand and use these. Consequently, this approach was abandoned and instead the answers were recorded verbatim and coded at a later date.

11.4.3 TR patients were asked four questions related to satisfaction:
a) How do you feel about the service you received from the ENT department?
b) How do you feel about the service you received from the H.A. department?
c) You waited ..... weeks/months for your ENT appointment after your doctor had written to the hospital. How did you feel about that wait?
d) You waited ..... weeks/months between seeing the ENT doctor and being fitted with your hearing aid. How did you feel about that wait?

11.4.4 DR patients were asked item (b), and items (c) and (d) amended to refer to the Hearing Aid Centre instead of ENT. Item (a) was only asked of those known to have been cross-referred to ENT and to have already been seen, but these were a very small minority. In addition, DR patients were asked an additional question: Was there anything that you were not satisfied with?

11.4.5 The verbatim answers to the questions about service and waiting times were dealt with in the following way. Lists of all the different answers received were drawn up, and each answer was rated by three judges, working independently, as to whether the statement was: 1) Very Positive 2) Positive

3) Neutral 4) Negative 5) Very Negative. The assessments of the three judges were compared, and where there was any disagreement the majority opinion, or failing a majority, the middle opinion, was accepted. With regard to the statements about service, the three judges agreed completely in 67% of cases, and in another 30% two agreed while the third put the statement in an adjacent category. In no case did one judge rate something as positive and another as negative. The results for the statements about waiting time were comparable: 62% complete agreement; 34% agreement within one category; and again no disagreements as to the side of the scale to use.

11.4.6 Examples of statements in each category are given in table 11.5. Quite a number of patients 'corrected themselves' when answering. For example, a frequent response was 'I thought the service was good – very good in fact'. In instances like this, the 'corrected' answer was taken. There were a few cases where a patient expressed praise for one aspect of the ser-

Table 11.5
Examples of statements from patients assigned to various categories of satisfaction

Statements about service received

Very positive:	Champion	First Class	Wonderful
	Excellent	Couldn't fault it	Perfect
	100%	Can't thank staff enough	Over the moon
Positive:	Good	Satisfactory	Quite happy
	Quite nice	Good attention	Pretty good
	Fine	Well treated	Efficient
Neutral:	Not Bad	No complaints	Can't grumble
	Adequate	O.K.	Alright
	Can't criticize	Reasonable	No problems
Negative:	Not very happy	Not satisfied	Disappointing
	Unsatisfactory	Staff not very helpful	Not happy
	Not what it was	It's too late to complain	
Very negative:	Disgusted	Staff couldn't care less	Big foul up
	Waste of time		

Statements about waiting time

Very positive:	Very pleased	Absolutely wonderful	Very short
	Very good	Splendid	Marvellous
	First class	Very quick	Excellent
Positive:	Good	No time at all	Pretty quick
	Fine	Quite satisfied	Not long
	Quite quick	Very acceptable	Fairly speedy
Neutral:	Normal	Haven't suffered	Not bad
	Didn't mind	Quite happy to wait	No bother
	Wasn't bad	Not too put out	Not that long
Negative:	Long time	Had to put up with it	Too long
	Jolly annoying	Seemed a long time	Not too good
	Not reasonable	Reconciled to waiting	Slow
Very negative:	Terrible	Very long time	Very annoyed
	Really disgusted	Fed up with waiting so long	Awful
	Damn long time	Diabolically slow	Shocked

vice, but was negative about another. In these cases, both ratings have been included in the analysis. There were also a number of replies which did not fit with any of the coding categories. This was more so with the waiting time items, where answers such as 'it was longer than I expected', or 'It was shorter than they told me' were quite common. For the purposes of the tables, these responses have been combined with the 'Neutral' category.

11.4.7 Table 11.6 summarizes the ratings of satisfaction with the service received. For TR patients this is the service from the ENT department at the appointment for an ENT examination. For DR patients it is the overall rating of the service from the Hearing Aid Centre. For both groups it became apparent that many patients could only rate the ENT doctor or technician they had seen, rather than the 'department' – particularly where this had been their only point of contact.

Table 11.6 Satisfaction with service received (figures are percentages of patients)

| | Traditional Referrals | | | | | Direct Referrals | | | | | Sample size | |
| | satisfaction with service from ENT | | | | | satisfaction with service from H.A.C. | | | | | | |
	V.Pos	Pos	Neutral	Neg	V.Neg	V.Pos	Pos	Neutral	Neg	V.Neg	TR	DR
Orange	56%	31%	–	13%	–			no data			16	nd
Red	47	18	35	–	–	71	18	12	–	–	17	17
Yellow	44	17	39	–	–	81	10	10	–	–	18	21
Green	57	33	10	10	–	86	–	14	–	–	21	14
Blue(NH)	59	29	6	6	–	100	–	0	–	–	17	17
Blue(PD)			not applicable			90	–	10	–	–	na	10
White	63	16	21	–	–	68	11	21	–	–	19	19
Black			no data			82	14	5	–	–	nd	22
Grey	35	15	20	15	20	74	11	11	–	5	20	19
Brown	80	13	7	7	–	85	5	10	–	–	15	20
Silver	82	18	–	–	–	95	5	–	–	–	22	21
Gold	61	22	17	–	–	89	11	–	–	–	18	18
Bronze	63	16	11	5	5	91	–	9	–	–	19	22
Overall*	59%	20%	16%	4%	3%	84%	7%	9%	0%	0.5%	186	188

*Overall figures based on Centres with TR and DR data only.
Note: figures can add to more than 100%

11.4.8 Both TR and DR patients showed fairly high levels of satisfaction, with very few patients of either group giving statements that were 'negative' or 'very negative'. Even so, there was a markedly higher level of satisfaction amongst DR patients than TR patients. In all Centres where comparable data was available, the proportion making 'very positive' statements was greater for DR patients. In some Centres, such as Yellow, Blue(NH), and Grey, the difference was quite dramatic. Over all comparable Centres combined, the proportion of patients making very positive statements was 59% for TR patients, and 84% for DR patients. The number of DR patients expressing negative comments was correspondingly lower: just 0.5%, compared to 7% of TR patients.

11.4.9 The question arises as to whether the difference in satisfaction levels could be due to factors other than the service received per se. The DR system was still relatively new when DR patients were interviewed and technician enthusiasm and interest may have still been exceptionally high. Also, nearly a year elapsed between the TR and DR interviews making it difficult to ensure that interviewer style remained constant. Some evidence that such factors do not explain the increased satisfaction under DR comes from the fact that TR patients themselves rated the service from Hearing Aid Centres higher than that from ENT: 71% were 'very positive' about this service, and just one negative comment was made. In addition, the result is supported by the objective findings that patients had shorter waits for their Hearing Aid Centre appointments, and were less likely to experience long delays in waiting rooms.

11.5 Patient satisfaction with waiting time
(tables 11.7 and 11.8)

11.5.1 Satisfaction ratings with the waiting time from GP referral to examination are presented in table 11.7. With regard to TR patients, the sample is somewhat reduced for this item. Apart from a few cases of missing data, the principal reason for this is that a proportion of those interviewed had not been referred by a GP, but had instead come from other hospital departments. In addition, there were some patients who could not remember who had referred them, and these were also excluded from this analysis.

Table 11.7   Satisfaction with wait for examination appointment (figures are percentages of patients)

	Traditional Referrals					Direct Referrals					Sample size	
	V.Pos	Pos	Neutral	Neg	V.Neg	V.Pos	Pos	Neutral	Neg	V.Neg	TR	DR
Orange	7%	26%	60%	7%	–			no data			15	nd
Red	6	6	50	33	6	–	13	81	6	–	18	16
Yellow	11	6	44	28	11	28	24	48	–	–	18	21
Green	6	17	65	6	6	36	21	29	14	–	17	14
Blue(NH)	13	6	62	13	6	41	35	24	–	–	16	17
Blue(PD)			not applicable			33	33	22	11	–	na	9
White	–	6	31	44	19	33	44	17	6	–	16	18
Black			no data			10	10	71	10	–	nd	21
Grey	–	6	82	6	6	21	32	26	11	11	17	19
Brown	14	7	71	7	–	39	22	33	6	–	14	18
Silver	11	11	42	32	5	33	33	33	–	–	19	21
Gold	6	6	76	12	–	28	39	33	–	–	17	18
Bronze	6	–	44	44	6	14	18	68	–	–	16	22
Overall*	7	7	57	23	7	27	28	40	4	1	168	184

*Overall figures based on Centres with TR and DR data only.

Table 11.8 Satisfaction with wait from examination to fitting (figures are percentages of patients)

	Traditional Referrals					Direct Referrals					Sample size	
	V.Pos	Pos	Neutral	Neg	V.Neg	V.Pos	Pos	Neutral	Neg	V.Neg	TR	DR
Orange	6%	33%	55%	6%	–	———————— no data ————————					18	nd
Red	11	11	67	11	–	–	23	59	12	6	18	17
Yellow	16	37	47	–	–	38	33	29	–	–	19	21
Green	10	37	53	–	–	46	31	23	–	–	19	13
Blue(NH)	5	5	67	17	5	12	41	47	–	–	18	17
Blue(PD)	———————— not applicable ————————					33	11	56	–	–	na	9
White	–	–	74	16	10	32	42	26	–	–	19	19
Black	———————— no data ————————					5	10	71	10	5	nd	21
Grey	–	39	44	6	17	29	12	47	12	–	18	17
Brown	10	25	55	5	10	35	30	35	–	–	20	20
Silver	29	10	57	5	–	38	38	24	–	–	21	21
Gold	16	16	68	–	–	28	33	39	–	–	19	18
Bronze	15	–	50	25	10	14	48	38	–	–	20	21
Overall*	12%	18%	58%	8%	5%	27%	34%	36%	2%	1%	191	184

*Overall figures based on Centres with TR and DR data only.

11.5.2 A high proportion of the responses to this item from both groups were neutral or non-committal, but despite this DR patients did show higher levels of satisfaction. This was so in all but one Centre (Red, where there was no difference). Overall, 55% of DR patients were positive, compared to just 14% of TR patients. This agrees with the factual finding, discussed elsewhere, that DR patients generally experienced considerably shorter waiting times.

11.5.3 The high proportions of neutral or non-committal answers concurs with observations by the interviewers that a high proportion of patients were very reluctant to criticize waiting times, even when the wait had been quite considerable. They tended to see their own requirements in relationship to those of other patients and to a health service they knew was under pressure. Thus answers such as 'My condition wasn't serious', 'other cases are more urgent', 'the service is overworked', and 'you expect to wait a long time these days', were frequently given.

11.5.4 With regard to the wait from examination to fitting of the aid (table 11.8), once again DR patients demonstrate higher levels of satisfaction, although the results are closer than for the previous satisfaction items. In terms of individual Centres, the proportion of DR patients expressing positive satisfaction is notably higher in 8 Centres, and about the same in 2 Centres. Overall (comparable Centres only) 61% of DR's gave positive statements, compared to 30% of TR's. Although there was a tendency for DR patients to experience a shorter wait between examination and fitting, the difference is probably not great enough by itself to explain the difference in satisfaction ratings. What seems more likely is that being generally more satisfied with other aspects of the service they have received, DR patients are more prepared to express satisfaction with this aspect as well.

11.6 Other aspects of service DR patients were not satisfied with

11.6.1 When asked if there was anything they were not satisfied with, the vast majority of DR patients replied in the negative. Many in fact were quite anxious to convey how pleased they were with the whole experience, particularly those who knew of people who had experienced long delays under the TR system. Just 9% (19 in all) mentioned things they had not found satisfactory.

11.6.2 The most common types of 'general' complaint were to do with the waiting time (4 patients) and dissatisfaction/problems with the aid (4 patients). Eight other patients made comments on specific things that had gone wrong for them. For example, two had been sent to the wrong hospital department (by the receptionist), where they had queued for some time before realising the mistake. Other such comments were about late hospital transport, delay in being seen on appointment day, not receiving the appointment card, etc. Perhaps of more interest was one complaint that there was no choice of NHS aids; the patient wanted an in-the- ear model. Another of relevance to the Centre concerned was that the department was badly situated for disabled people (it was on the first floor with no nearby lift).

11.6.3 Finally, there was some concern prior to the projects that patients would not be happy with being seen by a technician and not an ENT specialist. This would appear to be not so, as only one DR patient out of the 220 interviewed made a complaint of this nature. However, patients were not asked specifically about this, and it was also observed that a fair proportion thought that the technicians were doctors, principally because they wore white coats.

12 Impact of Direct Referral on the Job of the Technician

12.1 Introduction

12.1.1 The technicians and private dispensers who examined DR patients during the course of the project were each given a questionnaire to complete concerned with their experience of the schemes. The questionnaire was aimed at those below the level of principal audiologist or head of department. The private dispensers have been excluded from the results given in this section: they are discussed separately in a later chapter. Out of a possible total of 29 returns, 26 were received.

12.2 Impact on job satisfaction, workload, and service to patients
(table 12.1)

12.2.1 Presented with a list of items concerned with aspects of the job and the service received by patients, technicians were asked to rate each one as to how the situation during the main phase of DR compared to what it was like prior to DR. One technician had not been involved prior to DR, and therefore did not complete this section of the questionnaire.

12.2.2 With regard to items concerned with the job itself, the large majority of technicians rated most of these as being either 'better' or 'much better' than before. Particularly great improvement was noted with respect to job satisfaction (72% 'much better' or 'better'); the degree to which the job is interesting (72%); the variety of work involved (80%); and involvement with patients on an individual basis (60%). On none of these items did more than one technician rate the position as having got worse.

12.2.3 The only items where a substantial number rated the situation as worse were workload (28% 'worse than before') and stress (32%); although nobody rated any item as 'much worse than before'.

12.2.4 There were four items concerned with the service to patients. The great majority of technicians felt that DR patients received a better service than patients prior to the DR scheme (44% 'much better', 32% 'better'); though 2 technicians (8%) were of the opinion that it was worse. Both of these were from the same Centre. The position with regard to non-DR patients was more complex. While 20% felt this had improved, another 16% felt it had got worse. The four technicians who rated it as worse were spread across 3 different Centres.

12.2.5 There was a small number of technicians (24%) who felt that complaints from patients were less than before, and none who felt they had

Table 12.1
Technician ratings of job
under DR compared to
before pilot scheme
(figures in percentages)

Aspects of technicians job	Much better	Better	Same	Worse	Much worse	Don't know
The personal satisfaction you get from your job	32%	40%	28%	–	–	–
Your workload in relation to the time you have	–	16	52	28	–	4
The amount of responsibility that you are given	16	36	44	4	–	–
The degree to which you find the job interesting	28	44	28	–	–	–
Your personal relationship with the ENT department	–	8	88	–	–	4
The variety that the job provides	16	64	20	–	–	–
Involvement with patients on an individual basis	36	24	36	4	–	–
Your sense of being treated as a valued and respected hospital staff member	8	8	80	–	–	4
Degree of work-related stress	–	4	64	32	–	–
Aspects of service to patients						
The service that DR patients receive compared to the service patients received before DR	44	32	12	8	–	4
The service to non-DR patients	4	16	64	12	4	–
Number of patients complaining to you about any part of the service they have received	16	8	56	–	–	20
Your impression of the overall level of patient satisfaction	24	60	16	–	–	–

Note: All figures based on sample of 25 technicians.

increased; and a large number rated the overall level of patient satisfaction as higher under DR (24% 'much better', 60% 'better).

12.2.6 Technicians were also asked to write down any other aspects of the job or service they felt had got substantially better or substantially worse. Only three mentioned anything. One commented that the waiting list was shorter, while another noted that the wait for fitting that TR patients had was worse. The third comment was that being managed by the same person through the whole process from referral to fitting gave patients more confidence and better personal care.

12.3 Problems experienced by technicians seeing DR patients
(table 12.2)

12.3.1 The technicians were also asked to rate a list of possible problems they may have encountered. These could be rated as either 'Major', 'Minor', 'No Problem' or 'Don't know'. They were asked to do this separately for the early part of the project period and during the main phase of DR.

Table 12.2 Technician ratings of potential problems (figures in percentages)

	Early in the project				During main phase			
	Major problem	Minor problem	No problem	Don't know	Major problem	Minor problem	No problem	Don't know
The quality of direct referrals from GPs	31%	35%	31%	4%	15%	50%	35%	–
Additional workload	8	39	50	4	12	35	54	–
Confidence in your ability to examine DR patients	4	31	62	4	–	12	81	8
Number of DR patients needing a dewax	19	77	4	–	8	81	12	–
Your level of training	–	12	81	8	–	8	85	8
Your degree of experience	–	12	89	–	–	8	92	–
Your other work suffering as a result of DR	4	12	81	4	4	16	77	4
Obtaining advice from other audiology staff when you need it	–	8	92	–	–	4	96	–
Obtaining advice from ENT staff when you need it	12	15	73	–	4	19	73	4
Lack of ENT input on type of aid to be fitted	–	8	92	–	–	8	92	–

Note: All figures are based on sample of 26 technicians

12.3.2 In the early period, the main problems encountered were the quality of referrals (31% 'major problem'); the number of patients needing a dewax (19%); and getting advice from ENT when needed (12%). The additional workload was a major problem to 8%, and a minor problem to another 39%. One technician had a major problem with confidence in their ability to examine DR patients, and another 8 (31%) had a minor problem in this respect.

12.3.3 It is clear that the level of problems encountered diminished over the course of the projects: the total number of 'major problem' ratings declined from 20 for the early period to 11 for the main phase. The number experiencing major problems with the quality of referrals dropped from 31% to just 15%, and major problems with patients needing dewax fell from 19% to 8%. Both of these reductions were significant on the Wilcoxen test at the 5% level (two-tailed test). Those having major problems getting ENT advice also dropped, from 12% to 4%, but this reduction was not significant. The results also suggest a quite substantial improvement in levels of self-confidence, but again this did not quite reach significance.

12.3.4 On only two items was there any increase in the level of problems from the early period to the main phase. These were workload, and other work suffering due to concentration on DR. But the change is very minor (involving no more than one technician in each case) and nowhere near significant.

12.3.5 No technician mentioned any additional major problems which were not covered by the list presented.

12.4 Continuation of involvement in DR

12.4.1 The technicians were asked whether they would, personally, like to continue seeing DR patients after the end of the pilot project. Twenty-two (85%) answered yes, they would, while the remaining four were uncertain. None gave a categorical 'No'. This result indicates that, as a group, the technicians clearly felt that the benefits of DR outweighed the negative effects of the problems they had encountered. The principal reasons given for wanting to continue was that the DR system gave a faster, or better, service to patients. Eleven technicians mentioned these reasons. Three said they enjoyed the more personal contact with patients, and one liked the greater variety of work involved in DR. Two others simply said that the system 'worked well'.

12.4.2 Of the four technicians that were uncertain about continuing, two were so because of the level of poor quality referrals from the GPs. The other two were concerned about the increased workload with DR.

12.4.3 The technicians were also asked if they would like to see the DR system continue operating at their Centre after the pilot – irrespective of whether they personally wished to continue examining DR patients. Once again, the answers were very much in the affirmative, with 19 (73%) answering a straight 'Yes', and the remaining 7 answering 'Yes – with modification'. Again, no-one replied in the negative. With regard to the modifications they would like to see, the most common one, mentioned by five respondents, was that the quality of referrals from GPs would have to be improved, either by training GPs, changing the referral criteria, or making GPs take greater responsibility. Another modification, mentioned by two technicians, was that there should be ENT cover on the days that DR clinics are running, so that patients that need to be cross-referred can be seen the same day, and not have to make a separate appointment. One technician commented that there should be greater renumeration in line with the increased responsibility, and another wanted less time-consuming pro-formas.

12.5 Suggested improvements to the DR systems

12.5.1 In response to a question about practical ways in which their DR system could be improved, the area of greatest concern was the quality of GP referrals. Eight technicians suggested that increased communication with the GPs was needed, particularly with regard to giving feedback about the suitability or unsuitability of patients referred, and making sure GPs understood the referral criteria. Two others suggested that unsuitable patients should be sent back to their GP, rather than automatically cross-referred, to put some pressure on them to improve their practices.

12.5.2 The other major area needing improvement concerned ENT. Two technicians wanted ENT to take cross-referrals the same day, to reduce patient appointments, and two others wanted ENT advice to be more readily available.

12.5.3 All of the other suggested improvements were mentioned by single individuals, and most were very specific to their particular scheme. However, one technician suggested that referrals should be taken from sources other than GPs, such as health visitors, and another suggested that the system could be further speeded up if GPs could give hearing aid 'prescriptions', which patients would present at the Hearing Aid Centre.

13 Benefits, Problems and Disadvantages of the DR Schemes

13.1 Introduction

13.1.1 The head technicians and consultants that were interviewed were asked to complete checklists of potential benefits, problems, and disadvantages they may have experienced in running their DR schemes. The lists were different for the two groups, reflecting their different areas of experience. Head technicians were interviewed at all Centres, but consultants could only be seen at ten.

13.2 Benefits – head technicians
(table 13.1)

13.2.1 Head technicians were given a list of 8 benefits they may have experienced. Each of these could be rated as either 'Major', 'Minor', No Benefit', or 'Don't Know'. It became quite clear during the interviews that the great majority of head technicians were very enthusiastic about their DR schemes, and this is reflected in the number of 'Major Benefit' ratings given.

Table 13.1
Head technician ratings of benefits from pilot schemes (figures in number of Centres)

	Major benefit	Minor benefit	No benefit	Don't know
A faster service to patients	8	3	–	1
A better quality service to patients	10	2	–	–
Technicians have developed a more professional attitude to their job	7	4	1	–
Easier to develop community outreach services	1	4	5	2
More direct contact between the Hearing Aid Centre and GPs	7	4	1	–
Provides a more personal service to patients as individuals	6	4	2	–
Integrates the whole process of provision	8	4	–	–

13.2.2 The item 'A better quality of service to patients' was rated a 'Major benefit' by 10 of the 12 head technicians; 8 gave the same rating to 'A faster service to patients'; and the item 'Integrates the whole process of provision' also got 8 ratings as a major benefit. Only one item was not given 'major' ratings by a majority; this was 'Easier to develop community outreach services', but this is not surprising given that only a few Centres actively included a community provision element in their scheme.

13.3 Benefits – consultants
(table 13.2).

13.3.1 Nine out of the ten consultants interviewed gave a 'major benefit' rating to the item 'A faster service to hearing aid patients' (the last was a 'don't know'). Each of the other four items on the list was rated as either a major or minor benefit by at least half of the consultants.

Table 13.2
ENT consultant ratings of benefits from pilot schemes (figures in number of Centres)

	Major benefit	Minor benefit	No benefit	Don't know
A faster service to hearing aid patients	9	–	–	1
An improved service to other ENT patients	3	3	4	–
ENT time has been freed for more serious cases	2	7	1	–
ENT doctors have been relieved of seeing hearing aid patients they can do nothing for	3	3	4	–
Technicians have developed a more professional attitude to their work	3	2	3	2

NOTE: Consultants could only be interviewed at 10 Centres.

13.3.2 Perhaps one of the most important potential benefits of a Direct Referral system is that it can free up valuable ENT time. The item 'ENT time has been freed for more serious cases' addressed this issue; and although only 2 consultants rated this a major benefit, a further 7 gave it a 'minor benefit' rating. However, because under the pilot schemes all DR patients received an ENT safety-check, the full benefits of this would only have been felt after the pilot period. In the survey of pre-existing schemes this item was rated a major benefit by 62% of consultants, and a minor benefit by another 23% (Part II, section 33.7).

13.4 Problems – head technicians
(table 13.3)

13.4.1 Head technicians rated a list of 14 potential problems, both for the early part of the project and for the main phase. During the early period, the item with the most 'major problem' ratings referred to the number of patients being cross-referred to ENT: this was a major problem at 4 schemes (Orange, Yellow, Green, and Bronze), and a minor problem at another 4. Three other items were each major problems in the early days for three Centres: the quality of referrals (Green, Silver, and Bronze); having too few referrals (Yellow, Gold, Bronze); and funding the scheme (Yellow, White, Black). The quality of referrals was also a minor problem to another 5 Centres.

Table 13.3 Head technician ratings of problems (figures in number of Centres)

	Early in the project				During main phase			
	Major problem	Minor problem	No problem	Don't know	Major problem	Minor problem	No problem	Don't know
The quality of the direct referrals	3	5	3	1	2	6	4	–
Too many direct referrals	–	2	10	–	–	3	9	–
Too few direct referrals	3	3	6	–	1	2	9	–
Patient satisfaction with the scheme	1	–	9	2	1	2	8	1
Number of DR patients needing a dewax	2	5	4	1	1	7	4	–
Level of technician training or competence	–	2	9	1	–	1	10	1
Technicians opposing the DR scheme	–	1	11	–	–	–	12	–
ENT staff opposing the scheme	1	4	6	1	–	2	9	1
Funding the scheme	3	2	6	1	1	3	7	1
Day to day management of the scheme	2	5	5	–	2	3	7	–
Having staff to operate the scheme	2	2	8	–	1	3	8	–
General workload	2	4	6	–	1	4	7	–
The number of DR patients being cross-referred to ENT	4	4	4	–	3	5	4	–
Consultants 'off-loading' ENT referrals that mention 'hearing aid' or 'deafness' to the Hearing Aid Centre	–	5	7	–	–	4	8	–

13.4.2 Two other items, while not particularly major, received a high number of minor problem ratings: number of patients needing a dewax; and day-to-day management of the scheme. Interestingly, workload, which was one of the most important problems to the general technical staff seeing the bulk of DR patients, was not rated particularly highly by the heads of department.

13.4.3 On the whole, ratings for the main phase show a reduction in the number of major problems encountered. There was a total of 23 'major problem' ratings for the early period, compared with 13 for the main phase. This finding is in line with the results from the survey of general technical staff (section 12.3).

13.4.4 The single most important major problem continued to be the number of patients being cross-referred, which was still rated 'major' by Orange, Yellow, and Green, but was now only a minor problem at Bronze. With regard to quality of referrals, Silver reduced their problem, but it continued to be major at Green and Bronze. None of the Centres that were experiencing a major problem with too few referrals did so in the main phase, but it became major at a different Centre, Grey. Of the three Centres who initially experienced a serious problem with funding, only one, White, still did so during the main phase. There were a number of other instances, also, where major problems had been reduced or eliminated.

13.4.5 With regard to problems rated minor, the most important of these during the main phase were the number of patients needing a dewax, the quality of referrals, and the number being cross-referred. Finally, it is of interest to note that, contrary to some initial fears, no Centre at any time reported any serious problem with the number of Direct Referrals being too great.

13.4.6 Table 13.4 gives the number of problems rated as major for each Centre, for the early and main phases of the schemes. It can be seen that the majority, seven, of the Centres experienced no more than one major problem in either period. There were just two Centres – Yellow and Bronze – which initially had a large number of major problems, but both of these Centres had solved most of these by the time of the main phase. Overall, six Centres reported a lower number of major problems in the main phase compared to initially, while just two reported an increase.

Table 13.4
Number of benefits and problems rated by head technicians as major or minor

	No. of benefits (out of 7)		Probs–early period (out of 14)		Probs–main phase (out of 14)	
	Major	Minor	Major	Minor	Major	Minor
Orange	6	0	1	3	1	1
Red	2	3	–	–	–	–
Yellow	6	1	5	2	1	2
Green	1	4	2	5	2	5
Blue(NH)	5	1	1	7	1	7
White	6	0	1	7	–	9
Black	1	5	3	5	2	3
Grey	2	2	–	4	1	3
Brown	5	2	2	2	3	4
Silver	5	2	1	3	–	3
Gold	5	1	1	4	–	2
Bronze	3	4	6	2	2	6

13.5 Problems – consultants
(table 13.5)

13.5.1 The list of possible problems presented to consultants contained 6 items. With regard the early period of the projects, only one item received a 'major problem' rating: this was 'the number of patients being cross-referred to ENT', and this was rated as major by just one consultant, at Green. However, another 4 consultants rated this item as a minor problem. The same item was also on the list given to head technicians, and was the single most important problem according to them, as well. None of the other items received any 'major problem' ratings at all. However, 'not enough technicians' was given 4 'minor problem' ratings. Of the remaining items, two are of particular interest: 'Level of technician training or competence' received just 2 minor ratings, at Green and Black; and a question about the

Table 13.5 ENT consultant ratings of problems (figures in number of Centres)

	Early in the project				During main phase			
	Major problem	Minor problem	No problem	Don't know	Major problem	Minor problem	No problem	Don't know
Number of DR patients being sent to ENT for dewax	–	3	5	2	–	3	5	2
Level of technician training or competence	–	2	8	–	–	1	9	–
ENT staff opposing the scheme	–	1	9	–	–	–	10	–
The number of DR patients being cross-referred to ENT	1	4	5	–	1	4	5	–
Demands placed on service by DR system interfering with technician support for ENT clinics	–	–	9	1	–	1	8	1
Not enough technicians	–	4	4	2	–	4	4	2

Note: Consultants could only be interviewed at 10 Centres.

demands of DR interfering with technician support for ENT clinics was not rated as a problem by anybody.

13.5.2 With regard to problems during the main phase of the pilots, there was very little change from the early period. The consultant at Green still felt that there was a major problem with the number of patients being cross-referred to ENT, and the same four Centres were still having a minor problem with this. The minor problem with technician training at Black had been solved, but continued at Green; and a minor level of ENT opposition to the scheme at Gold had been resolved. In addition, a small amount of conflict developed at White between the demands of DR and of ENT clinics. There were no changes other than these.

13.6 Disadvantages – head technicians
(table 13.6)

13.6.1 Disadvantages were distinguished from problems by virtue of the fact that they tend to be factors which are inherent in a system, rather than difficulties which can be corrected. Only one of the listed disadvantages was given any 'major' ratings: this was the extra paperwork that DR generates for the Hearing Aid Centre (rated as major by 6 Centres). However, it is known that the data-collection involved in the evaluation was an onerous task for many Centres, and it is not clear whether respondents were distinguishing between this and the paperwork involved in DR per se when answering this question. It is true that DR does involve more paperwork than TR, but it may not be as large a disadvantage as this figure suggests.

13.6.2 Only two of the other potential disadvantages were given a notable number of negative ratings: that DR patients do not receive the benefit of ENT consultants advice; and that other aspects of the departments work have

Table 13.6
Head technician ratings of disadvantages (figures in number of Centres)

	Major disadvantage	Minor disadvantage	No disadvantage	Don't know
The extra paperwork generated for the Hearing Aid Centre	6	3	3	–
DR patients do not receive the benefit of the ENT consultants expertise	–	4	7	1
Loss of input from consultants on type of aid to be fitted	–	1	11	–
Service to non-DR patients has become poorer	–	–	12	–
Other aspects of Audiology Departments work have suffered due to concentration on DR	–	4	8	–
DR patients who would like to be examined by a doctor	–	2	8	2
Increased number of DNA's with DR	–	2	10	–

suffered due to concentration on DR. Both of these received 4 'minor disadvantage' ratings. Only one head technician felt that there was any disadvantage at all due to consultants not having any input on the type of aid to be fitted, and none believed that the service to non-DR patients had suffered at all.

13.7 Disadvantages – consultants
(table 13.7)

13.7.1 Presented with a list of 5 disadvantages they may have experienced with their DR schemes, consultants gave very few 'major' or 'minor' ratings. In fact, none of the issues received any 'major disadvantage' ratings

Table 13.7
ENT consultant ratings of disadvantages (figures are numbers of Centres)

	Major disadvantage	Minor disadvantage	No disadvantage	Don't know
DR patients do not receive the benefit of the ENT consultants expertise	–	3	7	–
Loss of input from consultants on type of aid to be fitted	–	3	7	–
ENT doctors are becoming distanced from hearing aid side of ENT work	–	3	7	–
Service to non-DR hearing aid patients has become poorer	–	–	10	–
Other aspects of Audiology Departments work have suffered due to concentration on DR	–	2	6	2

at all. The first three items on the list were to do with the involvement of ENT doctors with hearing aid patients: 'DR patients do not receive the benefit of the ENT consultants expertise'; 'Loss of input from consultants on type of aid to be fitted'; and 'ENT doctors are becoming distanced from the hearing aid side of ENT work'. Each of these received just 3 'minor disadvantage' ratings. However, it must be remembered that during the pilot schemes all DR patients received an ENT safety-check; and therefore the full impact of these potential disadvantages would not have been felt during the pilot period.

13.7.2 The question of whether DR will lead to ENT doctors becoming distanced from hearing aid work is particularly interesting. Consultants at the pre-existing schemes considered this to be the biggest disadvantage of DR: 15% rated it 'major' and 46% 'minor' (Part II, section 33.9).

14   Staff Opinions about the DR Schemes

14.1 Satisfaction with safety of the scheme

14.1.1 *Head Technicians*. When interviewed, most head technicians expressed a good to high degree of satisfaction with the safety of their DR schemes. There were just three that gave qualified answers. One felt that is was safe enough for elderly patients, but more doubtful for the young. During the pilot this Centre had been taking DR patients from 18 years of age upwards. Another answered by saying that at their Centre TR hearing aid patients were mainly seen by junior ENT doctors who 'have not the remotest interest in hearing aid patients and as a consequence I think the (TR) medical checks personally are a farce'. The third said that it was 'very safe but not absolutely safe' and was concerned that even a very small number of overlooked pathologies may not be an acceptable risk.

14.1.2 *Consultants*. On the whole, the consultants that were interviewed were even more positive about the safety of the schemes than the technicians. Nine out of the ten expressed very little doubt about the level of safety. Several gave high praise to their technicians, saying how good they were and how much confidence they had in them. A couple commented that it was 'at least as safe' as the TR system. The exception to this was one consultant who, although he did praise the work of the technicians as being 'excellent', nevertheless considered that all hearing aid patients should be seen by an ENT specialist and that anything else was a 'lowering of standards of patient care'.

14.1.3 *Other Safety-Check Doctors*. There was a bit more variety of opinion amongst the other 15 ENT doctors who were interviewed. Ten of these doctors considered that it would be satisfactory to operate the DR system without the safety-check element, compared to four who felt that all patients should continue to be seen by ENT (the remaining doctor was unsure). These four were divided across three different Centres.

14.1.4 In considering the above results, it should be borne in mind that doctors who were opposed to DR tended not to involve themselves in the pilots or to make themselves available for interview. Thus the above cannot claim to be a representative reflection of overall ENT opinion in these Centres. On the other hand, however, it is fairly representative of those who took an active part or an active interest in the schemes, and whose opinions, therefore, were at least informed by the practical experience of DR.

14.2 Desire to see the scheme continue

14.2.1 *Head Technicians.* Eleven of the twelve head technicians wanted to continue the schemes after the end of the pilot period. Some included a caveat, however, that this did depend upon a certain level of funding or staffing either being made available or being maintained. The principal reason given for wanting to continue was that DR provided a faster service to patients.

14.2.2 The head technician who did not want to continue was at Green. He did not reject DR entirely, but felt that a number of improvements would need to be made before it offered a satisfactory alternative to TR at his Centre. TR waiting times at Green were quite short, and therefore DR did not offer much of a benefit in this respect. The major problems with DR at this Centre that would need to be resolved were: 1) the large number of poor quality GP referrals, which led to an unacceptably high rate of cross-referral to ENT and increased likelihood that serious pathology might be missed. 2) technicians at this Centre had failed to identify significant pathology in a number of cases (the rate of non-crossed patients considered by ENT to require further management was the second highest in the study).

14.2.3 *Consultants.* As with head technicians, all of the consultants except for the one at Green wanted to continue the DR service. Some were very keen indeed: 'Yes, yes certainly would. Goodness yes. Oh! for goodness sake don't even suggest the opposite!'. Again like the technicians, the main reason for wishing to continue was because of the faster service to patients. Quite a number, however, also commented on the amount of ENT time that was freed for other patients.

14.2.4 The consultant at Green felt that DR had demonstrated no substantial benefits over the TR system, and he regarded it as in fact providing a lower standard of patient care. He also felt that Centres with long waiting lists would do better to run specialised ENT hearing aid clinics than to introduce Direct Referral.

14.3 Continuation, or otherwise, of schemes after the pilot period

14.3.1 At the time of interview many Centres, while wanting to continue DR, were unsure whether the scheme would continue or not. The Department of Health funding was coming to an end, and many places at that time did not know whether their health authority would take over the funding or not. There was subsequently a long period of uncertainty, during which some Centres were forced to suspend their schemes, and a number had to fight for continued funding.

14.3.2 Eventually however, most if not all of the difficulties were resolved, and Direct Referral systems were operating in all eleven of the Centres that wished to continue. We understand, however, that at least one scheme has run into funding problems since, and again been suspended. The twelfth Centre, Green, stopped DR completely. Apparently, however, at least one fund-holding GP practice has requested the Centre to restart, and they are considering implementing a limited scheme strictly for a small number of selected practices.

15   Cost Comparison of TR and DR

15.1 Introduction

15.1.1 The cost comparison of Direct Referral with the traditional system has been based on a 'bottom-up' approach. That is, costs have been calculated for each separate component of the two systems, rather than working from overall budgets. This was necessary because of the impossibility of separating out that component of an ENT budget spent on hearing aid patients as opposed to other patients.

15.1.2 A few of the projects involved private dispensers and/or community provision. The cost implications of both of these factors are considered later, in special sections. In the present analysis, any additional costs to DR arising from community provision have been excluded. With regard to the private dispensers, at two centres – Yellow and Brown – the dispenser worked alongside NHS technicians doing exactly the same job and being paid hourly, therefore they have been included in the costing of the DR system. The situation with respect to the other dispensers was rather different, and they have been excluded from the analysis in this section.

15.1.3 Two Centres – Red and Orange – are not included in the costing exercise due to the fact that not all of the necessary data was available from them.

15.2 Cost comparison for main site provision

15.2.1 The cost analysis covers the process of provision from a patients initial appointment with the GP, where referral is decided, up to and including the first follow-up after fitting. The analysis is done on the basis of computing the cost per patient fitted. It should be noted that no allowance has been made for resource wastage due to patients failing to attend appointments or dropping out of the process part way through. Most Centres slightly overbook to allow for the former and/or use the time to catch up on paperwork, and the latter are quite rare. This factor has been excluded because it differs very little between the two systems, and including it would add an unnecessary complication to the comparison of costs. At a rough guess however, resource wastage probably amounts to no more than 5% – 10% of overall costs, if that.

15.2.2 Another factor which is not considered in the following but deserves mention concerns additional expenditure which could be incurred if DR leads to an increase in demand for hearing aids. One Centre manager that we talked to estimated that something like 70% of his total expenditure was in fact consumed by the service to patients after fitting of the aid: in the form of follow-ups, repairs, repeat audiograms, replacement aids, tubing, batteries, etc. The reason why this proportion is so high is because patients come back for such services for many years subsequent to fitting. Consequently, if hearing aid fittings increase as a result of Direct Referral, there could be significant consequences for Centre costs in future years.

15.2.3 The various elements making up the service a patient receives under each system of provision are listed in figure 15.1. This figure is representative of the service received by the great majority of TR and DR patients. Costs, which will be presented later, have been computed for each element. Only direct costs – of salaries, materials, and instrumentation – have been included in the costing exercise. Indirect costs of operating the hospital as a unit have been excluded, the principal such elements being: capital costs, hospital management, hospital records, power, heating and lighting, building maintenance, catering, cleaning, laundry, security, telephone and mail systems.

15.2.4 The principal focus of the cost analysis is on the differential cost between the DR and TR systems, and the indirect costs will be assumed to be much the same for both systems: a Direct Referral patient may follow a different route of provision through the hospital system, but overall makes about the same demands on these indirect resources as a TR patient.

15.2.5 A number of minor factors which differ between the systems have not been included in the costing exercise. These are listed in appendix I.V.I. All of these factors are considered to have only very small cost implications, and because some relate to DR and some to TR, with regard to the differential cost they cancel each other out somewhat. In the main, these factors have been excluded either because of the difficulty of accurately costing them, or in order to simplify what is in reality a very complex situation.

15.2.6 Each of the projects went through an initial 'learning phase' when they first began seeing DR patients. It became clear that there were many factors, relevant to the costs of the system, which were different during this period. For instance, arrangements concerning which doctors would do the safety-checks, and when, took a while to organize properly. Also, the proportion of patients being cross-referred may have altered. It was also apparent from the data that technicians tended to take longer over the ear examination during the early period, and doctors longer over the safety-check. The intention of the costing exercise was to estimate a cost for DR operating 'routinely' – i.e. without the distortion of the initial learning process – therefore all of the analysis has been based on data from the second half of each project only. This also makes for a more valid comparison with the cost of the long-established TR system.

15.2.7 For each element in figure 15.1, a time or cost is given. These are based upon a variety of sources of information, though principally interviews and times recorded by staff while seeing DR and TR patients. Those elements of the provision process which are the same for both DR and TR, and carry the same cost, are printed in bold italics. The times or costs associated with these are therefore not critical with regard to the differential cost between DR and TR, though they obviously affect the overall cost of each system. It may be noted that the times spent by technicians on testing, impression taking, and fitting are given as the same for both systems, but have not been shaded. This is because the mix of grades of technicians who saw TR patients was different to the mix who saw DRs, and therefore the cost is different. Detailed reasons for each time or cost are presented in appendix I.V.II.

Figure 15.1
Components of TR and DR referral systems

TRADITIONAL REFERRAL		DIRECT REFERRAL	
GP Clinic		**GP Clinic**	
GP Clinic Time	5 min	GP Clinic Time	5–7 mins
First Appointment		**First Appointment**	
ENT Examination	7.1–11.1 mins	Technician Examination	11.2 mins
ENT doctor paperwork	3 mins		
Technician paperwork	5 mins	Technician paperwork	8 mins
Tech-Audio testing	14.8 mins	Tech-Audio testing	14.8 mins
Tech-Ear Impressions	9.3 mins	Tech-Ear Impressions	9.3 mins
ENT Clerical Officer	*15 mins*	*Audiology Clerical Officer*	*15 mins*
Audiology Clerical Officer	5 mins		
Impression Material	*£0.24*	*Impression Material*	*£0.24*
Audiology Instrumentation	*£0.10*	*Audiology Instrumentation*	*£0.10*
ENT Instrumentation	£0.10		
Fitting Appointment		**Fitting Appointment**	
Tech-Fitting	30.6 mins	Tech-Fitting	30.6 mins
Tech-Paperwork	*5 mins*	*Tech-Paperwork*	*5 mins*
Audiology Clerical Officer	*10 mins*	*Audiology Clerical Officer*	*10 mins*
Ear Mould	*£4.22*	*Ear Mould*	*£4.22*
Tubing	*£0.03*	*Tubing*	*£0.03*
Hearing aid	*£25.05*	*Hearing aid*	*£25.05*
Accessories	*£1.35*	*Accessories*	*£1.35*
Audiology Instrumentation	*£0.10*	*Audiology Instrumentation*	*£0.10*
Follow-up Appointment		**Follow-up Appointment**	
Technician time	*30 mins*	*Technician time*	*30 mins*
Audiology Clerical Officer	*10 mins*	*Audiology Clerical Officer*	*10 mins*
Audiology Instrumentation	*£0.10*	*Audiology Instrumentation*	*£0.10*
		DR Cross-Referrals Only	
		GP Clinic Time (only if re-referred by GP)	2–4 mins
		ENT examination	9.2 mins
		ENT doctor paperwork	3 mins
		Tech-paperwork	5 mins
		ENT Clerical Officer	10 mins
		Audiology Clerical Officer	5 mins
		ENT Instrumentation	£0.10

15.2.8 A mention needs to be made regarding the arrangements made by each Centre for managing DR patients cross-referred to ENT. After the end of the pilot projects arrangements changed at many Centres because it was no longer necessary for all patients to receive a safety-check. Costings are therefore based on the post-project arrangements. Cross-referred patients are now managed in one of two ways: they are either referred straight to ENT; or their GP is informed that they need an ENT appointment and is asked to re-refer.

15.2.9 Five Centres – Yellow, White, Black, Gold, and Bronze – cross-refer straight to ENT. At Gold however, an ENT consultant first looks through the technician reports and selects patients that need to be examined. Four Centres – Blue, Grey, Brown, and Silver – ask GPs to re-refer. The last Centre in this analysis, Green, abandoned DR and so the issue does not apply there. For the purposes of costing, however, Green has been taken as using each system 50% of the time. There is an additional expense involved in getting GPs to re-refer, which is principally the cost to the GP of producing and sending the re-referral letter (it is not necessary for the patient to go back to the GP).

15.2.10 The principal difference between the DR and TR systems is that under DR a technician screens the patients, whereas under TR they are seen by an ENT doctor. Consequently, the time that the technician spends with a patient compared to the time that an ENT doctor would have spent is a critical factor in the relative costs. In view of this, it is informative to take a closer look at the times involved prior to examining the costs attached.

15.2.11 The mean times taken by technicians and doctors over various procedures at each Centre appear in table 15.2. With regard to the technician examinations, it can be seen that the mean time ranges from a low of 6.4 minutes at Gold, to a high of 16.7 minutes at White. Both of these figures, however, are exceptional, as the rest are in the 9–13 minute bracket, with an overall mean of 11.2 minutes.

Table 15.2
Average times spent by technicians and ENT doctors with DR patients on various procedures (figures are in minutes)

	Technician examination	Audio testing	Ear impressions	Hearing aid fitting	ENT safety examination
Yellow	13.2 mins	12.2 mins	8.8 mins	37.7 mins	8.6 mins
Green	11.6	10.3	10.5	24.9	5.6
Blue(NH)	10.8	19.7	15.1	44.7	11.4
White	16.7	15.8	10.0	35.6	3.1
Black	9.0	13.3	7.4	37.2	8.8
Grey	10.9	16.4	5.0	26.4	4.4
Brown	(11.2)*	16.1	13.4	22.0	9.6
Silver	(11.2)*	21.2	10.0	28.0	5.7
Gold	6.4	11.8	6.2	22.4	5.0
Bronze	11.1	11.0	6.4	27.2	9.0
Mean	11.2	14.8	9.3	30.6	7.1

*Means could not be computed for these Centres, therefore the overall mean has been substituted

15.2.12 The mean times spent by ENT doctors on the safety-check vary from a low of 3.1 minutes at White up to 11.4 minutes at Blue, with an overall mean of 7.1 minutes. It was observed that 'local cultures' appear to exist with respect to the time taken: for example, all of the doctors at White recorded very low times for the examination, whereas at Blue and Brown they were all much higher. At least part of the difference between Centres in this respect can be explained by different attitudes regarding what the safety-check should consist of. Some doctors conducted a complete ENT examination, involving examination of the nose and throat as well as examining the ears and taking a history. Others felt that because these were hearing aid patients a history and check of the ears alone would suffice. A few doctors frequently recorded the time taken as being just 1 or 2 minutes (or even 30 seconds in a few cases!) which suggests that these doctors were often not even bothering to take a history, but just making a quick check of each ear for pathology.

15.2.13 Costings for the various elements of the two systems, for each individual Centre, are presented in tables 15.4, 15.5 and 15.6. With regard to salary costs, information was available concerning the grades of technicians and doctors who saw the patients. For each grade, the mid-point of the salary scale (from April 1991), including any superannuation and National Insurance, was used. This was then converted to an hourly rate working on the basis of a 37.5 hour week, and allowing for 10 days public holiday, 1 week sick leave, and four or five weeks holiday (depending on grade) per year. The details of the salaries and rates appear in table 15.3. London weighting has been applied where appropriate.

Table 15.3

Salaries and hourly rates for each staff grade

Salaries are as of April 1991. Hourly rates exclude holidays and sick leave

Grade	Salary (mid-scale point)	Hourly rate
ENT DOCTORS	£	£
Consultant	45,694	28.33
Senior Registrar	28,646	17.76
Clinical Assistant	28,646	17.76
Registrar	28,760	17.43
Senior House Officer	26,546	16.09
House Officer	20,096	12.18
TECHNICIANS		
MTO5	24,838	15.05
MTO4	20,369	12.34
MTO3	16,760	10.16
MTO2	15,757 (top of scale)	9.55
MTO2	13,319 (mid-scale)	8.07
MTO1	10,110	6.13
Student	6,892	4.18
CLERICAL		
Scale 2	7,587	4.50

London weighting: £1092 at April 1991, flat rate for all staff

Table 15.4 TR salary and material costs

SALARY COSTS (£s per patient)

	GP clinic 5mins	ENT exam low	ENT exam high	Audio test	Ear Imps	Aid fitting	3min Doc paperwork	10min Tech paperwork	15min ENT clerical	25min Aud clerical	30min MTO3 review	Total cost low	Total cost high
Yellow	4.44	2.31	3.38	1.74	1.27	4.60	0.80	1.36	1.13	1.87	5.08	24.60	25.67
Green	4.44	1.92	3.22	1.32	1.38	3.08	0.98	1.28	1.13	1.87	5.08	22.48	23.78
Blue	4.44	3.01	4.29	2.55	2.17	7.15	0.96	1.57	1.13	1.87	5.08	29.93	31.21
White	4.44	0.92	2.18	3.21	1.56	4.63	0.95	1.66	1.13	1.87	5.08	25.45	26.71
Black	4.50	3.19	4.66	2.53	1.47	7.39	1.09	1.96	1.29	2.15	5.41	30.98	32.45
Grey	4.44	2.00	3.82	2.60	0.82	4.10	1.37	1.59	1.13	1.87	5.08	25.00	26.82
Brown	4.44	3.19	4.67	2.54	2.03	5.93	1.10	1.84	1.13	1.87	5.08	29.15	30.63
Silver	4.44	3.57	5.07	3.08	1.69	4.59	1.12	1.69	1.13	1.87	5.08	28.26	29.76
Gold	4.44	1.95	3.37	2.02	1.05	3.76	1.07	1.71	1.13	1.87	5.08	24.08	25.50
Bronze	4.44	3.65	5.23	1.48	0.82	3.59	1.18	1.30	1.13	1.87	5.08	24.54	26.12
Mean	4.45	2.57	3.99	2.30	1.43	4.89	1.06	1.59	1.15	1.90	5.11	26.45	27.87

MATERIALS (£s per patient)

AUD Instrumentation	0.30	ENT Instrumentation	0.10
Impression Material	0.24	Mould and Tubing	4.25
Hearing Aid	25.05	Accessories	1.35

TOTAL MATERIALS COST = £31.29

Table 15.5 DR salary and material costs

SALARY COSTS (£s per patient)

	GP clinic 5min	7min	Tech exam	Audio test	Ear Imps	Aid fitting	13min Tech paperwork	35min Aud clerical	30min MTO3 review	Total salary cost low	high
Yellow	4.44	6.22	2.80	2.61	1.84	5.45	2.61	2.63	5.08	27.46	29.24
Green	4.44	6.22	1.99	1.76	1.80	3.26	2.10	2.63	5.08	23.06	24.84
Blue	4.44	6.22	1.86	3.38	2.54	7.15	2.18	2.63	5.08	29.26	31.04
White	4.44	6.22	2.91	2.76	1.75	6.15	2.27	2.63	5.08	27.99	29.77
Black	4.50	6.30	1.79	2.64	1.47	7.39	2.58	3.02	5.41	28.80	30.60
Grey	4.44	6.22	1.81	2.69	0.83	4.26	2.16	2.63	5.08	23.90	25.68
Brown	4.44	6.22	1.78	2.69	2.15	3.58	2.05	2.63	5.08	24.40	26.18
Silver	4.44	6.22	1.96	3.22	1.76	5.31	2.32	2.63	5.08	26.72	28.50
Gold	4.44	6.22	1.28	2.41	1.03	3.29	2.38	2.63	5.08	22.54	24.32
Bronze	4.44	6.22	2.36	2.29	1.36	3.20	2.31	2.63	5.08	23.67	25.45
Mean	4.45	6.23	2.05	2.66	1.66	4.90	2.29	2.67	5.11	25.78	27.57

MATERIAL COSTS

Instrumentation	0.30	Impression material	0.24
Mould and tubing	4.25	Hearing aid	25.05
Accessories	1.35		

TOTAL MATERIALS COST = £31.19

109

Table 15.6 Additional costs for DR cross-referrals

COSTS (£ per patient)

	GP clinic 2mins	4mins	ENT exam	3min Doc paperwork	5min Tech paperwork	10min ENT clerical	5min Aud clerical	ENT Instruments	Total cost	Percent crossed	Cost per DR patient
Yellow	na	na	2.44	0.80	1.11	0.75	0.38	0.10	5.58	45%	2.51
Green	1.78	3.55	2.79	0.98	0.85	0.75	0.38	0.10	6.74–7.63	34%	2.29–2.59 See (a)
Blue	1.78	3.55	3.68	0.92	0.86	0.75	0.38	0.10	8.47–10.24	14%	1.19–1.43
White	na	na	1.24	1.04	0.86	0.75	0.38	0.10	4.37	26%	1.14
Black	na	na	6.11	1.38	1.00	0.87	0.43	0.10	9.89	28%	2.77
Grey	1.78	3.55	2.96	0.85	0.83	0.75	0.38	0.10	7.65–9.42	7%	0.53–0.65
Brown	1.78	3.55	2.94	0.99	0.80	0.75	0.38	0.10	7.74–9.51	5%	0.38–0.47
Silver	1.78	3.55	2.56	0.90	0.87	0.75	0.38	0.10	7.34–9.11	11%	0.81–1.00
Gold	na	na	2.07	0.99	1.01	0.75	0.38	0.10	5.30	21%	1.24 See (b)
Bronze	na	na	3.09	0.88	1.10	0.75	0.38	0.10	6.30	4%	0.25
Mean	1.78	3.55	2.99	0.97	0.92	0.76	0.39	0.10			

Note: (a) Total cost and cost per DR patient based on assuming 50% of crosses go straight to ENT and 50% re-referred by GP.
(b) Another 26% of patients have technician exam results looked at by ENT consultant, but do not require examination, these have been costed in at 1 minute consultant time (equals £0.47 each).

15.2.14 It is important to note that the salary costs for each Centre take into account not only the grades of the technicians and doctors, but also the proportions of patients seen by each grade and the amount of time spent by different grades *in that Centre*. The details of how the costs were computed are given in appendix I.V.III. This approach yields the most accurate estimates of cost. It also preserves as much of the variability between Centres as possible, and this is particularly valuable when it comes to interpreting the overall results of the analysis.

15.2.15 For some elements of each system, the tables contain both a 'high' and 'low' figure. These are components which are important with regard to the differential costs between TR and DR, but for which an accurate single figure cannot be estimated. There are three such elements: the cost of the ENT examination for TR patients; the cost of the GP Clinic appointment for DR patients; and the additional GP clinic costs for DR patients who are re-referred to ENT. Many of the other costings are also not any more accurate, but have not been given a range either because they are small, or because they are the same for both systems and therefore do not have much influence on the *differential* cost between TR and DR. To give high and low costs for all of these would unnecessarily complicate the analysis.

15.2.16 Overall 'high' and 'low' costs for each system are presented in table 15.7. These figures are the sums of the individual component costs. The additional costs for cross-referred DR patients have been incorporated by expressing them as an average additional cost per patient fitted. It can be seen that, overall, the costs of the two systems appear quite similar, with the grand mean (over all Centres) for TR lying between £57.74 and £59.16, and that for DR between £58.29 and £60.16. However, given the approximate nature of the times used to estimate the costs of the GP Clinic, and of clerical work and paperwork, it would be wise to regard these figures as having an error attached of around plus or minus £5.

15.2.17 It appears from table 15.7 that the variation between Centres was fairly small, but because many components in the analysis were taken to be the same across all Centres – particularly the times spent on clerical work and paperwork, the GP clinic times, and the mix of aids fitted – the true degree of variation is undoubtedly under-represented.

15.2.18 Also given in table 15.7 are high and low figures for the *cost saving of DR over TR*. These figures can be regarded as being more accurate than those for the individual systems, as many of the more unreliable costs have been cancelled out in the subtraction. These figures suggest that TR is slightly less costly overall than DR (most of the savings are negative). There are three Centres – Yellow, Green, and White – where both the low and high differential costs are in favour of TR, one – Brown – where they both favour DR, and six where neither is favoured. The overall means suggest a range from TR being cheaper by £2.42 per patient, to DR being cheaper by £0.87.

Table 15.7 Total costs (salaries plus materials) for TR and DR (figures in pounds)

| | Traditional Ref. | | Direct Ref. | | Difference | | Diff using equal tech grades | |
	low	high	low	high	low	high	low	high
Yellow	55.89	56.96	61.16	62.94	−7.05	−4.20	−4.11	−1.26
Green	53.77	55.07	56.54	58.62	−4.85	−1.47	−3.47	−0.11
Blue	61.22	62.50	61.64	63.66	−2.44	0.86	−1.13	2.17
White	56.74	58.00	60.32	62.10	−5.36	−2.32	−4.01	−0.97
Black	62.27	63.74	62.76	64.56	−2.29	0.98	−2.16	1.11
Grey	56.29	58.11	55.62	57.52	−1.23	2.49	−0.90	2.82
Brown	60.44	61.92	55.97	57.84	2.60	5.95	0.26	3.61
Silver	59.55	61.05	58.72	60.69	−1.14	2.33	−0.12	3.35
Gold	55.37	56.79	54.97	56.75	−1.38	1.82	−1.36	1.84
Bronze	55.83	57.41	55.11	56.89	−1.06	2.30	0.38	3.74
Mean	57.74	59.16	58.29	60.16	−2.42	0.87	−1.66	1.63

Note: The 'low' difference corresponds to the lowest TR cost minus the highest DR cost.
The 'high' difference corresponds to the highest TR cost minus the lowest DR cost.

15.2.19 The above costings take into account the grades of technicians seeing DR and TR patients. DR patients are generally seen by senior staff, whereas juniors as well as seniors attend to TR patients, and this factor contributes to the figures suggesting that TR is slightly cheaper. In a practical situation, however, when a Hearing Aid Centre starts DR it may be able to reorganize the distribution of work in order to free seniors to see DRs without requiring any staff changes; for example, by ensuring that juniors take on a greater proportion of ENT clinic work, repair sessions, etc. Under these conditions the overall running costs of the department would not change, and therefore that part of the cost differential between TR and DR that is due to technician grades becomes more apparent than real (i.e. no actual increase in cost is experienced by the Centre). To represent this situation, high and low figures for the cost differential with the component due to technical staff grades removed are given in the final columns of table 15.7. In this case, the two systems appear very close indeed in cost, with the differential ranging from £1.66 in favour of TR, to £1.63 in favour of DR.

15.2.20 One factor influencing whether DR is cheaper than TR or not, is the proportion of DR patients who are cross-referred. The three Centres where both high and low differentials favoured TR all had high levels of cross-referral: Yellow (45% crossed), Green (34%), and White (26%). Conversely, those Centres where DR was most favoured had the lowest levels: Brown (5%), Bronze (4%). Nevertheless, the impact this has on the relative costs of the systems is not great.

15.2.21 It is of interest to examine how the overall cost of provision for each of the two systems breaks down in terms of GP, Hearing Aid Centre, and ENT components. These component costs are presented in table 15.8. GP clinic costs are a bit higher under DR; on average £5.48 per patient compared to £4.45. Not surprisingly, Hearing Aid Centre costs are the biggest element under both systems, the averages being £52.79 for DR, and £48.43 for TR. The extra cost here of DR is more or less equally matched by corresponding ENT savings, the cost of which drops from an average of £5.57 per patient under TR to £0.95 under DR. Prior to the pilot projects, there was some anticipation that Direct Referral might produce substantial ENT savings. However, these results show that, even under TR, ENT expenses represent less than 10% of the total cost of provision, and any savings here are balanced out by additional expenses elsewhere. One reason why ENT costs under TR are not greater is because a high proportion of patients are seen by the more junior ENT doctors.

Table 15.8 Breakdown of overall system costs by GP, Audiology, and ENT components (figures in pounds)

| | TRADITIONAL REFERRAL | | | | DIRECT REFERRAL | | | |
| | GP clinic | Hearing Aid Centre | ENT dept. | | GP clinic | | Hearing Aid Centre | ENT dept. |
			low	high	low	high		
Yellow	4.44	47.11	4.34	5.41	4.44	6.22	54.88	1.84
Green	4.44	45.20	4.13	5.43	4.74	6.82	50.23	1.57
Blue	4.44	51.58	5.20	6.48	4.69	6.72	56.19	0.76
White	4.44	49.20	3.10	4.36	4.44	6.22	55.07	0.81
Black	4.50	52.26	5.51	6.98	4.50	6.30	55.89	2.37
Grey	4.44	47.25	4.60	6.42	4.57	6.47	50.72	0.33
Brown	4.44	50.48	5.52	7.00	4.53	6.40	51.20	0.24
Silver	4.44	49.19	5.92	7.42	4.64	6.61	53.61	0.47
Gold	4.44	46.68	4.25	5.67	4.44	6.22	49.59	0.94
Bronze	4.44	45.33	6.06	7.64	4.44	6.22	50.48	0.19
Mean	4.45	48.43	4.86	6.28	4.54	6.42	52.79	0.95

15.2.22 The overall conclusion from this analysis must be that, on the whole, the cost differential between TR and DR per patient is very small, most likely no more than £2 either way. Slight alterations in the estimates for times taken over various procedures could alter the overall situation from one slightly in favour of TR, to one slightly in favour of DR. As a general rule, with a low level of cross-referrals DR is most likely to be cheaper, but as the proportion of crosses increases there comes a point at which TR becomes the most economic. Even with high rates of cross-referral, however, the cost difference between the systems is no more than a few pounds per patient.

15.3 Cost implications of community based DR schemes

15.3.1 There are two principal forms of community provision: domiciliary, where patients are examined and fitted in their own homes; and community clinics, undertaken at peripheral hospitals or health centres. There is an additional cost factor involved with community provision related to the times staff spend travelling and their travelling expenses.

15.3.2 Domiciliary visits are in general the more expensive type of community provision, because fewer patients are seen in one trip than at a community clinic. Unfortunately, the research did not yield rates for domiciliary visits, as the DR forms omitted to ask for information on where the patient was seen. Generally, however, the numbers of domiciliary visits are low (typically less than 5%), and our impression was that they did not vary greatly between the DR and TR systems – none of the head technicians gave any indication that domiciliary visits were a feature of their scheme.

15.3.3 It is useful, however, to have an idea of the additional cost of seeing somebody on a domiciliary basis. Nearly all of the technicians involved in community provision travelled by personal car (this was one of the questions asked of them), and the average distance that interviewed DR patients lived from the Centres was 5.5 miles. Therefore taking a figure of 11 miles for average distance travelled (there and back) on a domiciliary visit, requiring 22 minutes travelling time, this yields, for a mid-range MTO3, a salary cost of £1.85 and travelling expenses (at 33p per mile – NHS rate in 1991) of £3.63, which is £5.48 in total. Given that provision plus follow-up normally involves three journeys, this results in an extra cost of around £16 per domiciliary patient. However, it is usual for more than one domiciliary visit to be made on the same journey. If it is assumed that 3 patients are visited in the same trip, for a round journey of 20 miles, the extra cost (over 3 trips) reduces to about £10 per patient. These costs are probably much cheaper than transporting the patient and a carer to the Centre by ambulance or hospital car.

15.3.4 To see the same patient as a domiciliary under the TR system, however, would cost somewhat more. This would involve an ENT doctor making the first visit, with resulting higher salary costs. Furthermore, unless the doctor did the ear impressions, three technician visits would still be required, and so the overall cost would be considerably higher. In practice however, in many (if not most) cases where a TR patient needs to be seen as a domiciliary the ENT examination is waved, and the cost is exactly what it would be under DR.

15.3.5 Six Centres operated community DR clinics. At four of these however, prior to DR the ENT department were seeing TR patients at the same community sites, with technicians covering the clinics to do testing and impressions, and later fittings (at one, Grey, technician cover was suspended at the start of the pilot, but this was a temporary situation). The introduction of DR clinics at these sites therefore did not have any financial implications other than those covered in section 15.2.

15.3.6 The two Centres where community provision does have cost implications were Blue and Brown. The community DR service at Blue had two distinct elements. The first was NHS DR clinics at two locations. However, the situation regarding these was the same as that described above for other Centres, and they have no cost implications. The second element was community provision by a private dispenser. This is discussed in next section, which is devoted to the costs of involving dispensers.

15.3.7 The most radical change in community provision under the DR system occurred at Brown. Prior to the pilot there was a widespread system of community ENT clinics, but there was no technician cover for these, and all audiology work (including testing, impressions, and fitting) was done at the main site. Under the pilot scheme DR clinics were set up at six community sites. The distances from the main site were 14, 15, 16, 20, 22, and 25 miles. One technician covered each clinic, seeing an average of about 6 patients per clinic. No rent was paid for the rooms. On the basis of the technicians' grades, the approximate additional cost (salary and travelling over three trips) for the clinic 14 miles away works out at £8.58 per patient seen in the community, and for the clinic at 25 miles it is £15.31. The average over all 6 clinics is £11.43 per patient.

15.3.8 For information, the additional cost of operating a community clinic with a mid-range MTO3 seeing 6 patients per session works out at about 67 pence per patient served for each mile of distance (one-way) between the community clinic and the main site. Thus the additional cost of provision per patient for a community clinic situated 8 miles away would be 8 x 0.67 = £5.36. The patients themselves may make considerable savings in terms of travelling expenses and time.

15.4 Cost implications of private dispenser involvement

15.4.1 Private dispensers were involved at four projects. In two cases, however, the dispenser worked alongside NHS technicians doing exactly the same job and being paid an hourly rate. The only comparison relevant here, therefore, is their rate of pay compared to an NHS technician. At Yellow, the dispenser was paid £15 per hour, which is almost identical to the mid-point of the MTO5 scale, and worked there one day per week. At Brown, the dispenser was paid the same rate as a top-scale MTO2, and worked three days per week. Due to the manner in which these dispensers were employed, they have been included in the costings of the DR systems discussed in section 15.2.

15.4.2 The involvement of the dispenser at Grey was very different. The dispenser was, in fact, an employee of a private company, and was paid by them. The contract was between the company and the health authority. It has not been possible to determine the details of this contract. However, the evaluators were informed that the terms were quite favourable to the health authority, probably because the company was keen to be involved. The company pulled out of the contract half-way through the project, and the DR scheme was (after a brief period) taken on by the in-house NHS technicians. All of the costings for this Centre given in the previous section are based on the NHS technicians.

15.4.3 The final Centre where a dispenser was involved was Blue. Here the dispenser was self-employed and operated a scheme more-or-less independent of the NHS. The contract was that the dispenser was paid £45 plus VAT for each DR patient he saw. The costs of the hearing aid, earmould, and accessories were not included in this figure.

15.4.4 It is of interest to make a cost comparison between NHS provision and the private dispenser at Blue. However, the costs of NHS provision reported in previous sections have dealt with only the direct salary and material costs. In order to make the comparison valid , it is necessary to first estimate the contribution to NHS costs of the many indirect cost 'overheads', such as building costs, heating, lighting and power, maintenance, mail and telephone systems, etc.

15.4.5 The health authority has provided figures for 1991/92 expenditure for the Specialist Services Unit, of which ENT and the Hearing Aid Centre are part. The total salary costs were £41.15 million, non-salary costs were £12.61 million, and capital costs £9.23 million. The non-salary costs include heating, lighting, power, maintenance, drugs, medical consumables, station-ary, and various other items. Capital costs cover buildings, land, and equip-ment. Expressing the non-salary and capital costs as a percentage of salary costs, yields an approximate 'overheads' figure of 54%.

15.4.6 This figure is likely to be somewhat on the high side compared to the true overheads for hearing aid patients. These patients consume very little or nothing in terms of drugs, medical consumables, catering, laundry, and many of the other non-salary costs. The costs for 1991/92 for heating, lighting and power, and maintenance, on their own, were £3.35 million. Taking these plus capital costs as a percentage of salary costs produces a 'low' overheads figure of 31% of salary costs.

15.4.7 The direct salary costs to this Centre for each patient seen were £25.49 to £26.77 for a TR patient, and £25.74 for a DR. Taking £26 as the approximate average, the contribution of overheads, calculated at 31% and 54% of salaries, is between £8.06 and £14.04. This indicates that the total cost of NHS provision at this Centre (not including the aid) is somewhere between £34 and £40 per patient. Both of these figures are below the £45 plus VAT paid to the private dispenser. It is of interest to note that the head technician at this Centre came to regard the financial aspect of the dispensers involvement as unsatisfactory. The head technician reckoned that for the same outlay two full-time basic-grade technicians could have been employed, giving a total of 75 hours of work per week, in contrast to around 20 from the dispenser.

15.4.8 The overheads used above, however, do not take account of any *indirect salary costs*. There are many sources of indirect staff costs, includ-ing general hospital management, accounts and salaries, medical records, switchboard, mailroom, portering, security, maintenance, cleaning, laundry, catering, etc. Unfortunately, the figures available do not allow these to be distinguished from other salary costs. However, it is calculated that for indirect salary costs to make the total NHS cost greater than the amount per patient paid to the private dispenser, they would have to amount to somewhere between 13% and 32% of direct salaries and overheads (this assumes that the VAT paid to the dispenser is recovered: if not, the figures become 29% to 52% of direct salaries and overheads).

15.4.9 It is of interest to note that Brooks (1990) computed his estimate of overhead costs on a very different basis to the present analysis, but derived reasonable comparable figures. He computed two estimates. Firstly, on the basis of building costs over a 40 year mortgage period plus costs of rates, power, and janitorial services, he estimated a low figure of £10 per patient; and secondly, from information from private dispensers renting premises he computed a high figure of £20. These are not too far from the low and high estimates derived here, of £8 and £14.

16 Wax and Wax Removal

16.1 Arrangements made for dewaxing

16.1.1 A patient's ears need to be clear of wax before a reliable hearing test and proper examination can be carried out. GPs are normally expected to ensure that DR patients are free from wax prior to referral, but a number of DR patients still attend with obstructing wax.

16.1.2 A number of pilot Centres implemented a system whereby DR patients were requested to return to their GP shortly before attending the Centre so that he/she could ensure their ears were clear. This arrangement makes an extra GP visit for the patient. Even at these Centres, however, a number of patients still attended with significant amounts of wax.

16.1.3 There were three different types of arrangement in operation with regard to DR patients who were found to need wax removal upon presenting at the Centre: they were either sent back to their GP for a dewax; dewaxed at the hospital by an ENT doctor or staff nurse; or dewaxed by a technician. Only one Centre, Yellow, used the last form of arrangement. The other Centres were more or less evenly divided in terms of the system in operation, and some used a combination of both.

16.1.4 Each system has its pros and cons. Sending patients back to their GP makes, in many cases, two extra journeys for the patient (one to the GP, and one back to the hospital again), and delays their management. In addition, technicians complain that many GPs work to a different standard, and will regard an ear as clear which, from a technicians point of view, still has obstructing wax in it. On the other hand, sending patients back to their GP may encourage GPs to raise their standards, and make them more likely to ensure that ears are clean prior to referring. Therefore, while in the early stages of a DR scheme this arrangement may inconvenience some patients, this may be outweighed by the long-term benefits.

16.1.5 Where patients can be dewaxed at hospital, this has obvious advantages to the patient, particularly when it can be done the same day as their technician examination. Also the general standard of dewaxing is likely to be higher, making subsequent management easier. Against this however, is the drawback that this system provides no encouragement to GPs to improve their standards.

16.1.6 The last type of arrangement, training technicians themselves to dewax, is very controversial. Only two of the pilot Centres used this arrangement, and the evaluators have come across only two other Hearing Aid Centres in the country where it operates. The central issue is that this is a potentially dangerous procedure, but some technicians argue that if nurses can be trained to do it, there is no reason why they should not. Technicians involved in the pilot schemes were not asked directly if they would like to be trained to dewax, but when asked a general question about additional training, seven out of 26 specifically mentioned dewaxing. More information on the feelings of both technicians and ENT doctors towards this issue is provided in Part II.

16.2 Rates of DR patients attending with wax

16.2.1 The rates of DR patients attending with wax appear in table 17.1. At some Centres the rates were very high. Yellow had the highest at 37%. Two special factors may be contributing to this high rate however. Firstly, this Centre transferred long-waiting TR patients into the DR system; and secondly, technicians undertook dewaxing at this Centre, so GPs may not have been expected to dewax before referring.

16.2.2 There were notably high rates in two others places: Black (27%), and Gold (23%). With the exception of Blue(PD) all other Centres had rates between 8% and 17%. The private dispenser project at Blue did not report any patients attending with wax, but this result is highly suspect, as the NHS project at Blue recorded 15% attending with wax.

16.2.3 It needs to be noted that not all of those attending with wax were felt to require wax removal before management could proceed.

16.3 Wax removal (table 16.1).

16.3.1 The interviews with patients provided the most comprehensive data on wax removal. Patients were asked whether they had had any wax removed either at the GP's or at the hospital, from the day of referral onwards. In addition, the interviews also identified patients who had been dewaxed at the GP Clinic prior to the day of referral (GPs often do this to see if wax removal will improve hearing, and refer at a later date if it does not). The figures in table 16.1 include all patients dewaxed from the day of referral, or up to one year prior to the referral date.

16.3.2 Over all Centres for which data was available (nine in all), 46% of TR patients had wax removed, compared to 37% of DR patients. On a chi-squared test this difference is not significant (chi-square=2.96, df=1, p>0,05). These rates are really quite high, representing around two out of every five patients, and demonstrate how much of a nuisance wax must be.

16.3.3 The figures have been broken down into separate rates for the GP clinic and the hospital. GPs dewaxed 24% of TRs and 31% of DRs. This difference is not significant (chi-square=2.12, df=1, p>0.05). On the other hand, the proportions of patients being dewaxed at the hospital are markedly

Table 16.1   Percentages of TR and DR patients dewaxed

| | TRADITIONAL REFERRALS | | | DIRECT REFERRALS | | | Sample size | |
| | WHERE DEWAXED | | | WHERE DEWAXED | | | | |
	GP clinic	hospital	either	GP clinic	hospital	either	TR	DR
Orange	20%	27%	40%		— no data —		15	nd
Red	37	21	47	53	6	53	19	17
Yellow	10	40	45	19	19	38	20	21
Green	33	38	62	21	–	21	21	14
Blue(NH)		— no data —		76	–	76	nd	17
White	26	21	42	39	17	56	19	18
Black		— no data —		41	–	41	nd	22
Grey	5	19	24	37	5	42	21	19
Brown	30	10	35	21	5	26	20	19
Silver	23	54	68	38	5	38	22	21
Gold	20	25	40	28	6	33	20	18
Bronze	30	25	45	19	–	19	20	21
Overall*	24%	29%	46%	31%	7%	37%	182	167

*Overall figures based on Centres with TR *and* DR data only.

different: 29% of TR patients compared to just 7% of DRs (chi-square=27.7, df=1, p<0.001). Although this appears to represent a considerable saving of work for ENT staff, it will be seen later that this may be more apparent than real.

16.4 Failure to dewax

16.4.1 The figures given above reveal a marked drop, under DR, in the numbers being dewaxed at hospital, but no corresponding increase in wax removal by GPs. This might suggest that overall standards of wax removal decline under Direct Referral. This question has been examined using information from the examinations of TR and DR patients made by the external specialists (see chapter 10).

16.4.2 The two specialists recorded those cases where they felt wax removal was required, and the numbers of such patients can be compared for the DR and TR systems. These patients were all seen not very long after fitting, and represent cases where significant wax was present but not removed. The advantage of this data is that both sets of patients were examined by the same pair of specialists, which strengthens the power of the comparison.

16.4.3 Over all of the Centres visited combined, a total of 9 TR patients (out of 216) were identified as requiring wax removal; these represented 4.2% of the total. With regard to DR patients, 8 cases were found to need a dewax. However, another 3 DR patients had been discovered to have wax at the ENT safety-check, and had it removed previous to the specialist examination. These need to be added in, making a total of 11 cases with wax (out of 239), which was 4.6% of all DR patients. The TR and DR rates of failure to dewax, therefore, are almost identical.

16.4.4 This finding does not support the idea that dewax standards declined under DR. Therefore the fact that GPs did not dewax appreciably larger numbers of DR patients (even though the hospitals dewaxed fewer) would suggest that GPs were tending to send many patients with wax via the TR route, rather than remove it themselves. Consequently, the reduction in hospital wax removal work under DR is only apparent, as the patients with wax will turn up through the TR system instead.

17 GP Involvement and Referral Quality

17.1 Contacting the GPs

17.1.1 One of the initial tasks faced by the Centres when they implemented DR was to inform GPs of the scheme's existence. A number of Centres decided to start with only a section of GPs in their catchment area, either those from a particular region (Green, Gold, Bronze), or particular GP practices (Silver). The principal reason for this was concern about being 'flooded' with DR patients right at the start. The remaining Centres involved all GPs right from the start. In the event, concerns about 'flooding' proved to be unfounded, and the initial rates of referral were much slower than expected more-or-less everywhere. As a result, all of those Centres which had started with a restricted set of GPs fairly soon expanded the schemes to all practices.

17.1.2 All of the Centres except Red sent a letter to GPs informing them of the existence of the scheme and the referral criteria. (At Red, patients for DR were selected from the TR queue on the basis of the GP letter, and the Centre did not feel it necessary to inform GPs of the change.) The letters were in some cases sent directly, and in others distributed by the local Family Health Services Authority. Due to the initial poor take-up of the scheme, many Centres found it necessary to send further letters to encourage GPs to use it. It does not seem, however, that GPs in general were reluctant to use DR, but rather that they had not read or understood the content of the letter. At least one Centre had GPs whom they knew they had written to saying several months later that they had only just found out about the scheme.

17.1.3 In addition to letters, a number of Centres tried other means of disseminating information. Several offered to go out to GP practices and explain the scheme, but these offers were only occasionally taken up: there were only four such visits across all of the projects. One Centre arranged an open evening, but not one GP turned up. Others had considered the same idea, but knowing of the normally poor attendance at such functions, decided against it. At a couple of Centres, GPs who were found to be regularly sending patients eligible for DR via the TR route were contacted by phone. Finally, one Centre had a one-page spread about the scheme published in the local Trust Group magazine, which was circulated to all GPs.

17.1.4 Although slow to start, use of the schemes did build up over time at all Centres. This was partly due to the endeavours of Centre staff and partly to simple word-of-mouth amongst GPs. In a number of places, the latter led to some GPs who were strictly outside of the catchment areas referring patients, presumably in an attempt to circumvent long waiting lists in their own areas.

17.1.5 There was just one Centre, Red, which restricted the number of GPs using the system during the course of the project. Initially it was open to all, but at one stage the Centre wanted to set up a trial in which GPs would be audited. After this the scheme was more-or-less restricted to around 25 who agreed to take part.

17.1.6 All Centres with the exception of Red provided a set of referral criteria to GPs. At most Centres these were in the form of a checklist which the GP had to tick, and return with the referral letter. The only exception to this was at Yellow, where GPs were informed of the referral criteria in a letter, written by a consultant. An example of a referral checklist appears in appendix I.VII. In the main the checklists were based on the TTSA Direct Referral guidelines (appendix I.III). However, as a general rule, it was found that the more detailed the checklist, the more likely some GPs were to refer patients without ensuring that they matched it at all; and at least one Centre simplified and reduced their list part way through the pilot to try and improve the degree of compliance.

17.2 Frequency of GP use of DR schemes

17.2.1 It was anticipated from the start that not all GPs would wish to use Direct Referral. Also, for those who did, it is useful to have some idea how frequently it was used. To address these questions a detailed examination has been made of one Centre, Gold.

17.2.2 There were (according to the Centre) a total of 167 GPs in the catchment area. 117 of these (70% of the total) were represented among the 266 returns from this Centre. However, more GPs than this may have used the system, as forms were not returned for particularly inappropriate referrals. It appears therefore that the scheme did achieve a high degree of penetration into the local GP community over the pilot period. However, it should be noted that Gold did put considerable effort into making GPs aware of the scheme, and so this finding may not apply everywhere.

17.2.3 The numbers of referrals from individual GPs varied considerably. The maximum number from any one GP was 10, but this was exceptional: 51% of GPs made only one referral, and 81% made no more than 3. Given that the data spans nearly a full year of the DR system, it is calculated that the average referral rate per GP was a little over 2 patients per year.

17.2.4 The returns from other Centres have not been examined in such detail, but the impression obtained from a brief inspection was that the pattern was much the same, with the great majority of GPs making at most 2 or 3 referrals during the pilot year.

17.2.5 Given that use of the schemes build up slowly, it may be that many GPs did not start to use DR until well into the pilot period. The annual rate of referral per GP once the scheme has been running for a few years, therefore, may not be as low as these figures suggest. Stephens (1992) has provided comparable rates for two GP practices referring to a DR system which had been operating for several years. The GPs at one practice had an average rate of 6.3 patients per year, and at the other it was 3.2. These rates are still quite low, indicating on average one referral every two to four months.

17.2.6 Given that referral rates per GP are only low, it is perhaps not surprising that many appear to have a poor performance regarding the detection of ear pathology. This also raises the question of whether additional training for GPs in this area would have much impact when it would be called upon so infrequently.

17.3 Quality of referrals

17.3.1 The quality of direct referrals from GPs was one of the biggest problems for the pilot Centres. Three rated this a 'major' problem, and another five rated it 'minor' problem (see section 13.4). All Centres had their share of poor quality referrals. These ranged from things as obvious as patients who already had hearing aids or who were well below the age-criteria for DR, to more easily missable cases of ear disease, asymmetric loss, or conductive loss.

17.3.2 With regard to the most obvious factors that should have disqualified patients from being directly referred, technicians examining DRs were asked if they had personally come across any instances. All (26 individuals) had seen patients who needed dewaxing; 73% had seen people who had a hearing aid already; 36% came across individuals younger than the age criterion; 73% found 'obviously' discharging ears; and 74% saw patients with other 'obvious signs which the GP clearly should have noticed'.

17.3.3 An attempt has been made to estimate the rates of inappropriate referrals for each Centre (table 17.1). To do this, it has been assumed that any patient cross-referred to ENT by a technician can be considered an inappropriate GP referral. Also regarded as inappropriate are patients who attended with wax, or who already had a hearing aid. The figures must be regarded as only a rough guideline to the actual rates. Many Centres returned no forms for those who already had hearing aids, or for other particularly inappropriate patients, and so such cases are under-represented in the figures. (It is known, for example, that Green excluded 17% of referrals for such reasons, and returned forms for none of these.) Also, cases where the technician passed the patient but the safety-check doctor did not have not been included. On the other hand, a proportion of patients with wax did not present any management problems, so could pass as appropriate. Also, it may be incorrect to regard patients cross-referred *solely* for asymmetric or conductive loss as inappropriate referrals, given that GPs were not expected to conduct audiometry before referring.

Table 17.1 Inappropriate referrals (figures in percentages)

	Base Sample	Already had hearing aid	Attended with wax	Needed to be cross-referred	All types combined	All types combined 1st half	2nd half
Orange			DATA INCOMPLETE				
Red			DATA INCOMPLETE				
Yellow	246	No returns*	37%	38%	60%	52%	71%
Green	190	No returns*	9	28	35	31	39
Blue(NH)	278	No returns*	15	15	29	29	28
Blue(PD)	372	No returns*	0	3	3	2	4
White	398	5	8	24	32	29	35
Black	186	7	27	18	45	37	52
Grey	178	No returns*	17	13	29	30	27
Brown	304	5	9	5	19	18	20
Silver	311	2	11	9	19	19	18
Gold	266	No returns*	23	44	53	50	55
Bronze	183	6	12	7	24	28	20

*These Centres did not return forms for directly referred patients who already had hearing aids.

17.3.4 The figures in table 17.1 suggest that the rates of inappropriate referrals were generally pretty high. There is one low figure, of 3%, for the private dispenser project at Blue. In our opinion, however, this figure is very suspect: no forms were returned for patients who already had aids, no instances of patients with wax were recorded, and just 3% of patients were crossed. Given that these patients came from the same pool as those seen by the NHS project at Blue, which found 15% with wax, and crossed 15%, it seems most likely that the low rate is an artifact of the project management.

17.3.5 Excluding the Blue(PD) project, the rates of inappropriate referrals vary between 19%, at Brown and at Silver, and 60% at Yellow. Two other Centres had particularly high rates: Black (45%) and Gold (53%). In all, 7 (out of 11) projects had rates of over 25%. There are several unique factors which may have contributed to the very high rate at Yellow. Firstly, this was the Centre that transferred waiting TR patients into the DR scheme; secondly, it was one of the two places that did not require GPs to complete and return a criteria sheet; and thirdly, this was also the Centre where technicians carried out wax removal, and so GPs may not have been expected to remove wax before referring.

17.3.6 Despite caveats on the accuracy of our estimates, these results are comparable to the findings of others reported in the literature. Harries et al (1989) reported that of a sample of 100 TR patients referred specifically for a hearing aid, 46% failed the TTSA guidelines. In studies with equivalent patients, Campbell et al (1989) found 37% (out of 200 referrals) required further investigation or treatment; and Prinsley et al (1989) identified 19% needing same (out of 119). In none of the above, however, were GPs using a Direct Referral service. The one study which did involve DR was that of Hawthorne et al (1991), and here 56% of 225 DR patients were rated (by an

ENT surgeon) as unsuitable for Direct Referral. The variation in these results is wide, and in fact very similar to the range found amongst the pilot Centres.

17.3.7 As a test of whether GP referral practices improved over the course of time, separate rates have been computed for the first and second halves of each project (halves in terms of patients seen, not time). These rates (table 17.1) if anything suggest the converse: at most Centres they are higher in the second period, not lower. Particularly high increases were observed at Yellow (71% compared to 52% in the first half), and Black (52% compared to 37%). Given that cross-referrals by technicians represent a large component of the rates, it may be that this finding reflects a change in cross-referral practice rather than in the actual quality of referrals by GPs. This seems unlikely, however, in view of the fact that the finding is consistent across so many Centres.

17.3.8 A more likely explanation is that a high proportion of GPs referring in the second half had not used the scheme before, and were making much the same errors as earlier GPs. This is probable when it is considered that use of the schemes spread slowly, and that the great majority of GPs appear to have referred at most only 2 or 3 patients in the year (section 17.2). It may also be that the GPs who were first to use the schemes tended to be those with more interest in this field, which would explain a tendency for referral quality to be a little lower in the second half.

17.3.9 A somewhat different measure of referral quality is provided by the assessments of patients by external specialists and expert assessors (see chapter 10). On the basis of the experts' findings, we have estimated that towards the end of the pilot period around 24% of all patients showing (on their criteria) potentially serious conditions were being referred via DR, with the remaining 76% coming through TR (see appendix I.VI). In other words, GPs as a group appeared to be missing around one-quarter of all potentially serious abnormalities. This finding makes it quite clear that the inappropriate referrals are not just cases of trivial conditions.

17.3.10 It should not be concluded from the high rates of poor referrals that all GPs are poor at identifying appropriate cases for DR and ignore referral guidelines. Many Centres commented that they knew numbers of GPs who were excellent, and most GPs seemed willing to amend their mistakes once they were pointed out. However, there were a number of 'persistent offenders' who continued to refer inappropriate cases despite several attempts to get them to follow the criteria. In addition, when talking to patients, several Centres discovered cases where GPs had referred without even seeing the patient themselves, and others where a practice nurse made the referral.

17.3.11 Centres tried various ways of encouraging GPs to improve their practices. Many adopted the policy of writing back to the GP, explaining clearly why a particular referral was inappropriate, and with persistent offenders contact by telephone was sometimes tried. Particularly where a failure to dewax was concerned, a number (e.g Black, Grey, Silver) adopted the policy of sending all such patients back to the GP for wax removal. The effect of such measures over the course of the pilot period, however, appears to have been only small: towards the end of the period head technicians at two Centres still rated quality of referrals as a major problem (compared to three before), and six rated it as minor (compared to five before).

17.3.12 It may be, however, that referral quality will improve in the long term. The survey of pre-existing DR schemes, most of which had been running for several years, also addressed this issue. The percentage of head technicians who considered referral quality to currently be a problem was 35%, whereas 68% thought that it had been a problem in the past (Part II, section 33.3).

17.3.13 Nevertheless, the evidence is that GPs as a group make substantial numbers of inappropriate referrals, and a good proportion of these involve non-trivial conditions. Given this, it is clear that DR systems must place reliance upon technicians to detect significant ear disease and not solely upon the referring GPs.

18 Involvement of the Private Sector

18.1 Forms of involvement

18.1.1 There were four private dispensers involved in projects, each at a different Centre. The forms of involvement varied, and are described on an individual basis below. (Note: some of the dispensers were female, but all are referred to as 'he' to preserve confidentiality).

18.1.2 *The Dispenser at Yellow*. The private dispenser involved here was well known to the Centre, and they had been recommending him to patients who wanted to buy a private aid for several years. He had been working as a dispenser for over 10 years. During the pilot project, the dispenser worked alongside the NHS technicians doing a more or less identical job. He was employed by the Centre for one day a week, and was paid an hourly rate, equivalent to the mid-point of an MTO5.

18.1.3 *The Dispenser at Brown*. This dispenser had 25 years post-qualifying experience, and had also worked within the NHS for 3 years. As with the dispenser at Yellow, he was working alongside NHS technicians and doing exactly the same job. For some time he had been working at the Centre 3 days a week, being paid an hourly rate equivalent to a top-of-the-scale MTO2.

18.1.4 *The Dispenser at Grey*. The private dispenser involvement at Grey was on a very different basis to those previously discussed. He was an employee of a private company, and the contract was between the company and the hospital. The dispenser had 11 years post-qualifying experience, and had been with the company for 2 years. The intention was that the Direct Referral project would be run entirely by the dispenser, at two peripheral sites, without the involvement of NHS technicians. The project was slow to get off the ground, and after it had been running for about 6 months, came to a halt. The company terminated the contract with the hospital. The precise reasons for these actions are not clear. The consultant said that there were difficulties in the general relationship between themselves and the company, partly due to a clash of cultures and partly because of lack of previous experience.

18.1.5 *The Dispenser at Blue*. At Blue, the private dispenser and the NHS Hearing Aid Centre ran largely independent projects. Although the dispenser had not worked with the Centre previously, he was well known to them, and had been working as a dispenser for 22 years. All patients were directly referred to the Hearing Aid Centre, but these were then 'shared out' between themselves and the dispenser. The dispenser saw patients in private dispensing rooms at two different locations, and made his own appointments with them. The Centre paid him £45 + VAT for each patient he served.

18.2 Performance of the private dispensers

18.2.1 The performance of private dispensers relative to NHS technicians at the same Centres will be examined on three counts: in terms of proportions of patients for whom a dewax was arranged; proportions cross-referred to ENT; and the numbers of cases with potentially serious pathology that were missed.

18.2.2 *Dewaxing.* There was very little difference between dispensers and NHS technicians with regard to rates of patients deemed to require wax removal. The highest rates were at Yellow: 22% for the dispenser and 21% for NHS staff. At Grey the rates were 13% compared to 7% respectively; at Brown 2% compared to 4%; and Blue 0% as against 2%. The only difference that was statistically significant was at Blue (Chi-square with Yates correction = 5.95, $p < 0.05$). This Centre arranged for the great majority of patients to be dewaxed by GPs before attending, but there must be some concern that out of over 350 patients the dispenser considered none to require wax removal.

18.2.3 *Cross-referral.* At two Centres dispensers demonstrated a significantly lower rate of cross-referral: at Yellow it was just 4% compared to 47% for NHS staff; and at Blue it was 3% compared to 15%. In both cases the difference is significant on a chi-square test at the 1% level. These results suggest that the dispensers were not cross-referring all the patients they should. At Brown, although not significantly different, the rates suggest that NHS technicians here were also more likely to cross-refer: 6% as against 2% by the dispenser. At Grey both dispenser and NHS staff had the same rate, 13%.

18.2.4 *Potentially Serious Pathology.* Amongst the patients examined by private dispensers there were four cases of potentially serious pathology picked up by local ENT doctors that had not been cross-referred. Three of these failures were committed by the same dispenser, and this was more than by any other individual in the study.

18.2.5 With regard to the sample of DR patients examined by the external specialists, 35 of these had originally been seen by dispensers, but only one case was considered (by the specialist) to need anything more than a hearing aid, and this was for a non-serious condition. Therefore this data has nothing to contribute to assessment of the performance of the dispensers.

18.3 Opinions about the dispensers' involvement

18.3.1 At two Centres both the head technician and the dispenser themselves appeared to be quite satisfied with the outcome of the latters involvement. Both dispensers said they would like to continue seeing DR patients after the end of the pilot. One felt that his involvement had given him more confidence in his own abilities and decisions, and that this would help in his private work as a dispenser. The only comments the other made were that, from a personal point of view his involvement had been 'quite successful', and that there was a greater degree of satisfaction in having seen a patient through the entire provision process, compared to the TR system.

18.3.2 At the remaining two Centres technicians reported a number of problems with the performance of the dispensers. At one of these there were a number of instances where technicians identified potential pathology missed by the dispenser. They also considered that his history taking was very inadequate, and the standard of audiometry poor and in many cases insufficient. Also, in one case the head technician felt that the dispenser had incorrectly recommended a commercial aid to a patient – although due to lack of knowledge about NHS aids rather than anything else. On the plus side, technicians acknowledged that the great majority of patients seen by the dispenser were very pleased with the service he gave.

18.3.3 The dispenser himself felt that from his point of view the involvement had been very successful and he had found it interesting. However, he did not consider it a financial success. Even so, he was keen to continue under a different arrangement.

18.3.4 The remaining Hearing Aid Centre was also not happy with the work of the dispenser there. Apparently there was a lot of problems with him mixing up earmoulds and prescription forms, losing moulds, and so on. The head technician said they were still sorting out the mess several months after the project had come to an end. The dispenser himself did not comment on his involvement.

19 Community Provision

19.1 Introduction

19.1.1 There have been suggestions that it is easier to arrange for community provision of hearing aids within a Direct Referral framework. Community provision within the traditional system generally requires the involvement of both an ENT doctor and a technician, whereas under Direct Referral the technician alone can run a clinic or see a patient in their own home. It has also been suggested that technicians may be more prepared to take their work into the community than some doctors.

19.2 Community provision within the pilot schemes
(table 19.1)

19.2.1 The principal forms of community provision are clinics run at peripheral hospitals or health centres, and domiciliary visits. In addition, there may be visits to old peoples homes, day centres, adult training centres, hostels, and – fairly rare – clinics run at GP surgeries. The various types of site where directly referred patients were seen under the pilot projects are summarized in table 19.1.

Table 19.1 Locations at which DR patients were seen during pilot schemes

	Main hospital site	Peripheral hospitals/health centres	Domiciliary visits	Old peoples' homes	Other locations
Orange	Yes	–	–	–	–
Red	Yes	–	Yes	Yes	–
Yellow	Yes	Yes	Yes	Yes	–
Green	Yes	–	–	–	–
Blue(NH)	Yes	Yes	–	–	–
Blue(PD)	–	–	Yes	Yes	Private dispensing rooms
White	Yes	Yes	Yes	Yes	–
Black	Yes	–	Yes	Yes	Old peoples' day centre
Grey	–	Yes	Yes	–	–
Brown	Yes	Yes	Yes	Yes	GP surgery
Silver	Yes	–	Yes	Yes	–
Gold	Yes	Yes (Inpatients only)	Yes	Yes	–
Bronze	Yes	–	–	–	–

19.2.2 With regard to domiciliary visits, nine of the projects undertook these within the context of the Direct Referral system. Reliable figures for the proportions of DR patients seen as domiciliaries are unfortunately not available, but it is known that at all Centres they were only a very small percentage.

19.2.3 Six Centres operated DR clinics at peripheral hospitals or health centres (at Gold, however, the peripheral hospital clinic was for inpatients only). In the great majority of instances, however, the sites involved had operated community *ENT* clinics prior to DR, and so the DR clinics did not represent a spreading of community provision, though they probably did mean that more patients could be seen in local situations. One of the conditions of being a pilot site was that all DR patients should receive an ENT safety-check, and it is possible that this factor was responsible for most DR clinics being restricted to such places. Another factor was that many of these community ENT clinics had developed long waiting lists, and in many cases the DR clinics were set up at these sites specifically to try and reduce these.

19.2.4 There were just two Centres where the peripheral clinics represented a more involved change to the service than the above. These are considered individually below.

19.2.5 BROWN. At this Centre, the ENT clinic system prior to DR was already heavily community orientated. The health authority covers a large area, and ENT clinics were run at a good number of peripheral sites, with something like 86% of new hearing aid patients coming from these, and 14% from the main hospital. There was no technician cover at the community ENT clinics, and so the audio test and impressions could not be done on the same day as the ENT examination. Instead, patients had to travel some considerable distance to the main hospital for these, and then again at a later date for fitting.

19.2.6 DR clinics were organised at those community sites experiencing the longest waiting lists. Six sites were involved, at distances ranging from 14 to 25 miles from the main Centre. The DR clinics meant that patients could be fitted within two appointments as opposed to three, and that the whole process could be undertaken at a local site.

19.2.7 BLUE. Prior to DR, hearing aid patients were seen at three peripheral sites, as well as at the main base. A team of ENT doctors and technicians serviced these peripheral clinics, and so the entire provision process could be conducted locally, normally in two appointments. As part of the pilot DR scheme, a private dispenser conducted additional community clinics at two other sites. There was one difficulty, in that the premises involved were upstairs rooms and some disabled patients were not able to take advantage of being seen locally. However, the private dispenser also did a number of domiciliary visits. The NHS technicians themselves operated community DR clinics at two of the sites where community ENT clinics were conducted. Plans for a third site did not come to fruition. Towards the end of the project period, however, these NHS operated community DR clinics had to be halted. The difficulty was that the hospital group was seeking Trust status, and use of the rooms was going to have to be re-negotiated.

20 The Impact of Hospital Trusts and Fund-Holding GPs on Direct Referral

20.1 During the pilot period

20.1.1 During the pilot projects, the cost of serving DR patients was met almost entirely from the Department of Health funds each Centre received to run the schemes, and therefore the emergence of fund-holding GPs, and the adoption of Trust status by participating hospitals, had very little effect on the DR systems at this time.

20.1.2 At the start of the pilot projects there was only one participating hospital seeking Trust status. Since then, quite a number have become Trusts or are currently seeking Trust status: Orange, Red, Yellow, Green, Blue, White, Grey, Brown and Gold.

20.2 Developments since the end of the pilot period

20.2.1 In the period since the pilot schemes ended, one very significant consequence of the new funding arrangements has emerged. This concerns the fact that fund-holding GPs pay a different cost depending on whether they refer a patient to ENT or to a Hearing Aid Centre. The figures vary greatly from one place to another, but a typical price for an ENT appointment may be in the region of £50-£100. This compares to a Hearing Aid Centre appointment cost of typically half this sum. This makes Direct Referral very economical for fund-holding GPs. It was shown in section 15 that the actual costs of the two systems are not all that different (even excluding the GP costs), and so from the point of view of a Trust hospital, DR is far less profitable than TR.

20.2.2 This factor has caused a number of complications with regard to DR patients that need to be cross-referred to ENT. In order to ensure that the GP pays for the ENT appointment, a number of Centres now require that the patient be re-referred to ENT by the GP themselves, rather than crossed directly by the technician. Four of the pilot Centres introduced this system subsequent to the end of the project, although it is not known whether there were other considerations as well as the financial one guiding this decision. This arrangement causes extra inconvenience to both the GP and the patient. Although the latter does not have to personally return to the GP in order to be re-referred, it does mean that they cannot be seen in ENT the same day that they saw the technician.

20.2.3 It has also become apparent that in some areas the hearing aid/audiology service, and particularly DR, has not been given appropriate consideration by Trust financial managers when computing charges. At least part of this failure is due to the fact that Audiology Units have historically been subsumed within the ENT department. At Centre Brown, for example, the health authority set a cost for audiology appointments for 1992, but excluded the cost of the hearing aids fitted. Consequently, in order to avoid a substantial financial loss on DR patients, this Centre maintained the arrangement of all DR patients receiving an ENT safety-check long after the end of the pilot period, so that GPs could be charged for an ENT appointment.

20.2.4 The move to Trust status has also had some consequences for community provision. At least one Centre had to suspend community DR clinics while it renegotiated the use of rooms at community sites, following a move to Trust status. During the pilot period none of the Centres was paying rent for the use of rooms in community locations. It may be that this will change under the new arrangements, particularly where the Hearing Aid Centre is in one Trust and the community sites in another. The same thing presumably applies to community ENT clinics.

20.2.5 One final observation to be made is that many fund-holding GPs appear to be keen on Direct Referral systems. Centre Green, which abandoned DR after the pilot, has had requests from fund-holding GP practices that they restart it. Also, the evaluators have heard of a number of instances where non-pilot Centres have received requests from fund-holders that they start a Direct Referral scheme. At least part of the motivation behind this may be the relative cheapness (to the fund-holder) of sending a patient via Direct Referral.

21 Effects of Direct Referral on Demand

21.1 The question of demand

21.1.1 A question of interest is whether Direct Referral systems have any impact on the amount of demand for hearing aids. If there are substantial demand implications, then this may have important consequences in terms of the staffing levels required to keep up with demand, and the overall costs of the service.

21.1.2 To answer this question adequately – at least with regard to the pilot projects – information would be required on the numbers of patients (TR and DR) that GPs referred for hearing aids, both over the pilot period and for some period previous to that. Unfortunately, such data is not available. Figures for total outpatient referrals to ENT departments are available for some Centres, but these do not distinguish hearing aid patients from other types, and there is no way of separating them out. Data on audiometric tests conducted and hearing aids fitted has been obtained, but the numbers of these are determined principally by staffing levels: an increase in the GP referral rate would increase the length of waiting lists, but without additional staff would not be reflected in an increase in tests or fittings.

21.1.3 Head technicians were asked if they felt that demand had increased since the start of the project: 7 answered 'Yes', 3 answered 'No' and the remaining 2 could not say. However, amongst those who said 'Yes', only 3 were confident that DR had been a factor in this. It is worth noting that regular GP health-checks for the over-75's were introduced just before the start of the projects, and this could well have had an impact on demand.

21.1.4 The evidence from the pilots is that use of the DR schemes by GPs spread fairly slowly, and was still in a process of expansion at the end of the pilot period. Given this, any impact of DR on overall referral rates was probably only small over this period. A number of Centres provided data on numbers of first-time hearing aid fittings done, both during the project and for some time preceding (table 21.1), and this can be used to examine in more detail the degree of use that GPs made of the DR systems.

21.1.5 Firstly, it is worth noting that (for the seven Centres for which figures are available) the statistics on first-time fittings do not suggest any large increase between 1990 and 1991 (when the DR schemes got fully under way): the total fittings over all Centres in 1990 was 8,566, and in 1991 it was 9,247, an increase of only 8%. In addition, while 4 Centres show an increase

Table 21.1

Departmental statistics on numbers of first-time hearing aid fittings

	1987	1988	1989	1990	1991
Orange	*	*	667	*	*
Red	*	*	*	1612	1594
Green	*	*	*	1581	1464 (approx)
White	*	*	929	850	1321
Brown	*	*	1016	1306	1432 (approx)
Silver	*	771	819	848	810
Gold	1419	1334	1262	1339	1463
Bronze	*	*	*	1030	1163
Total				8566	9247

*=No data

between these two years another 3 show a decrease, and where there is several years' data there is quite a lot of fluctuation over time. These results simply bear out what was said previously: that numbers of fittings depend more on variations in staffing levels than anything else.

21.1.6 For six Centres that provided first-time fittings information on a monthly basis, the proportion of all hearing aid fittings that were DR patients has been computed. This has been done for the 'middle' six months of each project. The early months were excluded because these tended to be a 'run-in' period when very few DRs were seen and the schemes were just getting off the ground. The last two to three months have been dropped because the numbers of forms returned for this period was unrepresentative (many DR fittings in this period were not part of the pilot sample – inclusion in the sample was usually based on date of first appointment).

21.1.7 The resulting percentages appear in table 21.2. All DR patients who did not go on to be fitted with an aid have been excluded (including those who already had aids). At three Centres (White, Brown and Silver) the proportion of fittings that were DRs was over 30%; at Gold it was 27%; at Green 18%; and at Red 10%. The low proportion for Red is due to the Centre restricting the number of GP practices using the DR scheme (see section 17.1).

Table 21.2

First-time fittings that were DR patients

	Number of first-time fits in 'middle' six months of pilot	Number that were DR patients	Percentage DR
Red	599	62	10%
Green	724	131	18%
White	709	239	34%
Brown	559	189	34%
Silver	384	150	39%
Gold	742	197	27%
Total	3717	968	26%

21.1.8 In table 21.3, the data has been summed across all Centres (excepting Red, see above) on a periodic basis to illustrate the growth in DR fittings over time. This analysis covers all fittings over the first nine to ten months of each project. In the earliest period 14% of all first-time fittings were DR patients, and this rises fairly steadily over time, at a rate of approximately 3% per month, until in the last month 36% were DRs. The rate of increase is quite slow, and there is no suggestion of levelling off towards the end. What this data cannot tell us, however, is how much of this shift to DR provision is due to an increase in GP referral rates, and how much to GPs directly referring patients they would otherwise have sent via the TR route.

Table 21.3

Trend in Direct Referral fittings over time (Centre red excluded)

	Number of first-time fits	Number that were DR	Percentage DR
'Early' period	1822	254	14%
First (subsequent) month	553	109	20%
Second month	544	138	25%
Third month	655	168	26%
Fourth month	459	128	28%
Fifth month	491	153	31%
Sixth month	519	158	30%
Seventh month	450	161	36%

21.1.9 Although the question regarding demand cannot be completely answered – other than to say that any influence during the pilot period was probably small – the proportion of fittings that were DR in the final period (36%) and the fact that the rate of growth was not slowing does suggest that at this point there was still room for continuing expansion of DR provision.

21.1.10 Despite the lack of hard evidence, however, there are a number of good theoretical reasons for expecting Direct Referral to lead to an increase in demand, and these are discussed in section 22. However, it may take longer than the year that the pilots ran for any effect on demand to reach an appreciable level.

22   Direct Referral and Rehabilitation

22.1 Audiological rehabilitation

22.1.1 Audiological rehabilitation refers to the total process by which a hearing-impaired patient is helped to be able to communicate optimally, given his sensory deficit, and to minimise the handicap experienced (Stephens, 1983, p284). It is important to note that rehabilitation does not stop at the fitting of a hearing aid. Indeed, this is very much only a first step – albeit a very important one – in the rehabilitation process. The aid may be of little value unless the patient learns to make the best use of it, and may need to be supplemented by other measures, such training in lip-reading, help with tinnitus, and the use of environmental aids (e.g. special doorbells, telephone attachments, etc).

22.1.2 In the context of comparing the TR and DR systems, the important issues are: a) what effect, if any, does the system of provision have upon the likelihood of a hearing-impaired individual seeking help; and b) what effect does it have upon the rehabilitation process subsequent to hearing aid fitting. In particular, does the DR system enhance or diminish either of these elements.

22.2 Direct Referral schemes and patient motivation to seek help

22.2.1 Although no hard data is available, there are several good reasons for believing that Direct Referral is likely, if anything, to encourage people with a hearing deficit to seek help, and at the very least will not deter it.

22.2.2 Stephens (1983) identifies seven classes of factors influencing the likelihood of a hearing-impaired person seeking rehabilitative help: physical status; psychological status; social factors; educational and vocational factors; accessibility of the services; attitude of professionals encountered; and experiential factors. It is with respect to the last three classes that Direct Referral procedures are likely to have a beneficial influence.

22.2.3 *Accessibility*. There are two principal ways in which DR can improve accessibility. Firstly, by removing the referral to an ENT consultant the system is simplified (at least for the majority who are not cross-referred) and speeded up. This removes some factors which might have deterred individuals with only low or moderate motivation. For example, in our interviews with DR patients it became apparent that a number had not sought help previously because they had heard of waiting times of a year or more, and had not considered it worthwhile to enter the system.

22.2.4 Secondly, if DR makes it easier to develop community based pro-vision, in terms of patients being served at community clinics or where they live, then geographical accessibility will be enhanced. This would be particu-larly important in rural areas where the main site may be far away and public transport poor, and also important to the disabled.

22.2.5 The development of community provision was limited under the pilot schemes, principally because of the requirement that all patients have an ENT safety-check. However, in the survey of pre-existing schemes 53% of Centres rated the development of outreach services as a major benefit of their DR system, and another 21% rated it a minor benefit (Part II, section 33.6). A note of caution must be sounded here, however, as where there are community clinics without ENT cover there may be a temptation not to cross-refer patients who really need to be seen by an ENT surgeon, particularly if this means the patient making a trip to the main site.

22.2.6 *Attitude of professionals.* The principal groups of professionals involved in hearing aid provision are GPs, ENT doctors, and audiological technicians. With regard to GPs, DR can have some beneficial effects on attitude. If a GP finds that patients he has directly referred have been dealt with faster and have found the whole experience generally more pleasant, then he may be more likely to recommend referral to other hearing-impaired patients. Several of the pilot Centres commented that they had received letters from GPs praising the DR service.

22.2.7 Again, however, there must be some note of caution, as it may be that some GPs find that a large proportion of the patients they directly refer are deemed inappropriate by the Hearing Aid Centre, and are referred straight back to them. In some cases this could make the GP disillusioned not only with the DR system, but with the hearing aid service in general.

22.2.8 With regard to the attitude of technicians, it is quite clear from the research that a high majority derive a great deal of job satisfaction from seeing patients within a DR framework (section 12.2). This must make many patients feel that they are being managed by people who are highly motiv-ated and genuinely concerned with their wellbeing. Certainly the great majority of DR patients interviewed were very pleased with the service they had received, and many praised the technicians highly.

22.2.9 *Experiential factors.* The degree of motivation that a person has for seeking help is heavily influenced by the experiences of others known to him who have been through the process. The shorter waiting times and higher levels of satisfaction found amongst DR patients can therefore be expected to increase the motivation of other hearing-impaired individuals. Indeed, a number of the DR patients interviewed said they approached their GP because they had friends or spouses who had had good experience of the DR system and received their aid quickly.

22.3 Influence of DR on post-fitting rehabilitation

22.3.1 While there are good reasons for believing that DR systems can increase the probability that hearing-impaired individuals will seek rehabilitation help, the issue of what happens subsequent to the fitting of an aid is another question altogether. The importance of this phase of the rehabilitation process should not be underestimated. For example, Ward (1980) estimated that something like one-third of patients fitted under the NHS with hearing aids give up using them after only a short period. This percentage may have declined since his study, due to the spread of follow-up systems, but may still be high. A substantial waste of resources is implied when patients give up the aid purely because of a lack of motivation or support subsequent to fitting.

22.3.2 Unfortunately, the present research is severely limited with regard to what it can say about the post-fitting rehabilitation process. No hard data pertaining to this has been generated, although some attempts were made.

22.3.3 It has been reported in another section (3.3) that the initial patient interviews were conducted at the review appointment and attempted to collect data pertaining to rehabilitation, but that this did not succeed due to the high proportion of patients who did not return for their follow-up. Subsequent interviews were done at fitting.

22.3.4 An attempt was also made to collect information about aftercare by including a section on the DR data forms indicating whether the patient had been referred on to a hearing therapist, social worker, or voluntary visitor. Unfortunately, the information provided was very scarce, presumably because time constraints forced us to limit data collection up to the point of fitting, and decisions on such referrals are often taken at a later date to this. Consequently this data has not been reported.

22.4 Arrangements for post-fitting rehabilitation

22.4.1 Although data related to post-fitting rehabilitation is not available for individual patients, information is available on the arrangements at each Centre concerning this.

22.4.2 Seven Centres employed no hearing therapists, though one (Green) had a vacancy for one (this was at the start of the project, it may have been filled since). One Centre, Gold, had a half-time hearing therapist. The remaining four places – Black, Grey, Brown, and Bronze – each employed two hearing therapists. No information is available, however, on the degree of involvement of the therapists with hearing aid patients.

22.4.3 With regard to the arrangements made to follow-up patients subsequent to fitting, there were two places (Grey and Silver) where no formal follow-ups were done, though patients were free to return if they had problems. The problem at both of these Centres was that they did not have the technical staff to cope with reviewing all patients. One other Centre did not do follow-ups at the start, but has implemented a scheme since. This is in fact operated by Hearing Therapy, who review patients once at the hospital, and then once at home.

22.4.4 All of the other Centres except for Red provided just one formal follow-up appointment to each patient. In addition, Blue ran quite a comprehensive voluntary visitor system in which all patients were offered the chance of being visited at home; and three other Centres (White, Black, and Gold) did a number of home visits. Red operated what appeared to be the most thorough rehabilitation system. This was the only Centre to conduct two formal follow-ups, and they also operated a voluntary visitor system. In addition, this Centre used a checklist to assess each patient's requirements in terms of environmental aids, training in lipreading, tinnitus advice, and so on.

22.4.5 The central issue in the present context is whether DR is in any way beneficial or detrimental to this phase of rehabilitation. There are several features which can be seen as beneficial. If the experience has been pleasant, a patient having difficulties may be more willing to return for further assistance. Provision in the local community might further enhance this. Also, in most places DR patients are managed by the same technician throughout the provision process, and this means that there is a key individual familiar with the particular problems of each patient that they can turn to. Lastly, where domiciliary visits are involved the technician is in a position to make a good assessment of a patients needs with regard to environmental aids.

22.4.6 On the negative side, however, it may be that a patient's motivation to persevere with the hearing aid is related to the personal 'cost' involved in obtaining it: generally speaking, the higher the cost, the greater the motivation (because the perceived degree of loss implied in giving up is greater). Thus if the aid has been obtained in a short time with little difficulty, the patient may undervalue it and have less incentive to overcome any difficulties experienced in learning to use it. This may be particularly true of those patients who right at the start had low motivation and only entered the provision system initially because it looked 'easy'. If the easy accessibility of DR systems attracts large numbers of such patients, at the end of the day the end result could be a greater, instead of smaller, waste of resources.

23   Medico-legal Responsibility

23.1 Introduction

23.1.1 The legal position regarding Direct Referral, if something were to go wrong and a patient begin litigation proceedings, is not clear-cut (RNID 1989). It is certainly not safe to assume that the technician involved would automatically be 'covered'.

23.1.2 Under the traditional system the legal situation is fairly straight-forward (Baguley et al 1989). The ENT consultant to whom the patient was referred has examined the patient and decided that a hearing aid was the most appropriate form of management. If this is later questioned, the notes of the examination are available, and the consultant would take formal responsibility for any negligence. The Medical Defence Union would then defend any suit. The same applies if the patient had been examined by a less senior doctor working under the orders of the consultant.

23.1.3 With Direct Referral the position is more complex. Both the GP and the technician apply a set of criteria which had previously been agreed with the ENT consultant. If an underlying serious pathology were missed it is not certain who would be considered to be responsible. If the condition were one that obviously contradicted the criteria provided to the GP, then the GP would most likely take responsibility. If the condition were more subtle, how-ever, or not covered by the criteria for GPs (which are often less detailed than those followed by technicians), then the technician is in an awkward position. The GP could argue that he followed the criteria and is therefore not responsible, and the consultant never examined the patient, and therefore did not have the opportunity to make a correct diagnosis. The technician would then be exposed to a possible claim, particularly if the criteria were not correctly followed. Furthermore, it is not clear to what degree the employing health authority might accept liability for the technician's action (Baguley et al 1989).

23.2 Arrangements at the pilot Centres

23.2.1 During the pilot period, medical responsibility was not really an issue for participating Centres. This was because all DR patients were given an ENT safety-check, and therefore the consultants took responsibility. How-ever, where schemes were continuing after the pilot period – without the safety-check element – head technicians and consultants were asked about the arrangements they had made regarding responsibility. Opinions differed with some believing the GP would be responsible, and some the consultant.

Just one head technician thought that they personally would be the responsible party. No Centre had, however, done anything to formally establish what the position would be.

23.2.2 These results mirror very closely the findings for the pre-existing DR schemes (see Part II, section 31). Of the 21 schemes visited in that survey, only one had gone into the issue in any real depth. This Centre asked the health authority's solicitors to examine the question. The outcome of this was an acknowledgement of shared responsibility between the GP and consultant.

23.2.3 The GP is responsible inasmuch as he/she needs to ensure that the referral is an appropriate one. The consultant is viewed as being responsible for ensuring that the technical staff are adequately trained and that the practice is safe. He therefore takes medical responsibility for the actions of the technical staff that he has trained and evaluated. If however a technician was shown to have acted in a negligent fashion, for example by flouting the set criteria, then that technician could be held to be personally or jointly liable.

23.2.4 Arranging legal cover for technicians

23.2.5 Given that in certain circumstances technicians may find themselves liable, it is sensible to ensure that they have legal cover for their DR work. There are two ways of achieving this. The first is personal indemnity insurance, as is already used by some private dispensers (RNID 1989).

23.2.6 The second, and probably preferable, approach is to ensure that the health authority will accept liability. The Centre mentioned above found that the health authority takes liability for the actions of their staff *provided those actions fall within the remit of their job description*. It seems likely that the same would apply elsewhere. This Centre therefore ensured that the management of DR patients was specified in each senior technicians job description. This was done in the form of a letter from the health authority. It should be noted that although this ensures that if there is any litigation, at the end of the day the authority will be the body that pays out, depending on circumstances they themselves could take action against the technician involved.

Appendix I.I

Pro-formas used to collect data on DR patients

Appendix I.I.I: Patient Details Form
Appendix I.I.II: Technician Examination Form
Appendix I.I.III: ENT Doctor Examination Form

Direct GP Referral Pilot Project

Direct Referral Record Sheet

Hospital _____

Patient Details

Name _____   Hospital no. _____

Sex: ☐ Male ☐ Female   Age _____

Referred by: ☐ GP ☐ Other   Date of referral letter _____

GPs' name _____   GP's address _____

Wax

Only complete this section if patient attends with significant wax

☐ Dewaxed today at hospital

☐ Wax does not prevent action on this patient

☐ Will return for dewax   Todays date _____

☐ Sent back to GP for dewax   Time spent _____ (mins)

Audiometric Testing

AC	☐ 1ear	☐ 2ears	ULLs	☐ 1ear	☐ 2ears
BC Unmasked	☐ 1ear	☐ 2ears	Tympanometry	☐ 1ear	☐ 2ears
BC Masked	☐ Yes		ARTs	☐ 1ear	☐ 2ears

Other _____

Hearing level in better ear: 0.5k _____   1k _____   2k _____   4k _____

Time spent with patient _____ (mins)

Initials _____   Date _____

Audiologist/Technician Examination

Please complete separate examination sheet, but only after any wax problems have been resolved

Ear Impressions

Time spent with patient _____ (mins)

Initials _____   Date _____

Aid Fitting

If no aid was required, tick here ☐

Aid fitted: B.E _____   B.W _____   Commercial _____

Ear: ☐ Left ☐ Right ☐ Bilateral

Time spent with patient _____ (mins)

Initials _____   Date _____

Aftercare

☐ Hearing Therapist   ☐ Voluntary Visitor   ☐ Social Worker

Other _____

Direct GP Referral Pilot Project

Audiologist/Technician Examination

Hospital _____

Patient name: _____ Hospital/Patient no. _____

Findings of History and Examination

S = Significant reason for cross-referring patient/seeking ENT advice.
P = Present but not significant.

Sudden Onset of Loss _____ ☐ S ☐ P

Fluctuating Loss _____ ☐ S ☐ P

Loss in one ear Only _____ ☐ S ☐ P

Vertigo _____ ☐ S ☐ P

	Right ear			Left ear	
☐ S	☐ P	___ Earache _____	☐ S	☐ P
☐ S	☐ P	___ Tinnitus _____	☐ S	☐ P
☐ S	☐ P	___ History of Discharge ___	☐ S	☐ P
☐ S	☐ P	___ Active Discharge _____	☐ S	☐ P
☐ S	☐ P	___ Diseased Canal _____	☐ S	☐ P
☐ S	☐ P	___ Perforation _____	☐ S	☐ P
☐ S	☐ P	___ Inflamed Drum _____	☐ S	☐ P
☐ S	☐ P	___ Scarred Drum _____	☐ S	☐ P

Findings of Audiometry

☐ Significant Asymmetric Loss   ☐ Significant Conductive Loss

---

Other significant reasons

Action

Tick all that apply

☐ Degree of loss does not warrant Hearing Aid

☐ Appropriate to fit Hearing Aid

☐ Cross-refer to ENT (ENSURE REASONS ARE TICKED OR WRITTEN ABOVE)

☐ Review patient's ears again at later date

☐ Other _____

Was input of another staff required in making exam/decision? ☐ Yes ☐ No

IF YES: Who _____

IF YES: How much of their time _____ (mins)

Time spent with patient _____ (mins)

Initials: _____   Date: _____

** NOW STORE THIS SHEET SEPARATELY FROM THE OTHER PATIENT NOTES **

Direct GP Referral Pilot Project

ENT Doctor Examination

Hospital _____

Patient name: _____ Hospital/Patient no. _____

Findings of History and Examination

S = Significant factor prompting further investigation/intervention.
P = Present but not significant.

Sudden Onset of Loss _____	☐ S	☐ P
Fluctuating Loss _____	☐ S	☐ P
Loss in one ear Only _____	☐ S	☐ P
Vertigo _____	☐ S	☐ P

Right ear			Left ear	
☐ S	☐ P ___ Earache _____		☐ S	☐ P
☐ S	☐ P ___ Tinnitus_____		☐ S	☐ P
☐ S	☐ P ___ History of Discharge__		☐ S	☐ P
☐ S	☐ P ___ Active Discharge_____		☐ S	☐ P
☐ S	☐ P ___ Diseased Canal_____		☐ S	☐ P
☐ S	☐ P ___ Perforation_____		☐ S	☐ P
☐ S	☐ P ___ Inflamed Drum_____		☐ S	☐ P
☐ S	☐ P ___ Scarred Drum_____		☐ S	☐ P

Findings of Audiometry

☐ Significant Asymmetric Loss   ☐ Significant Conductive Loss

---

Other significant factors (including conditions not to do with the ear)

Action

Tick all that apply

☐ Degree of loss does not warrant Hearing Aid
☐ Appropriate to fit Hearing Aid
☐ Further Investigation required (ENSURE FACTORS ARE TICKED/WRITTEN ABOVE)
☐ Medical Intervention required (ENSURE FACTORS ARE TICKED/WRITTEN ABOVE)
☐ Review patient's ears again at later date
☐ Other_____

If a specific medical condition has been identified, please specify _____

If treatable, how serious could the consequences be for this patient if this condition was not treated?

In near future:	☐ Not Serious	☐ Serious	☐ Very Serious	☐ Cannot tell
In long term:	☐ Not Serious	☐ Serious	☐ Very Serious	☐ Cannot tell

Comment_____

Time spent with patient_____ (mins)

Initials:_____ Date: _____

Appendix I.II

Pro-forma used by external specialists

Direct Referral Pilot Project

External Specialist Examinations: Patient Details Form

Hospital _____

***   **Please ensure that when he sees a patient, the specialist**   ***
***   **has this form (completed) together with the patient's**   ***
***   **audiogram and other relevant audio test results**   ***

Patient Name_____

Patient Hospital Number_____

Sex: ☐ Male   ☐ Female

Age _____

Aid Fitted _____

Date on which Patient was last Examined _____
(Date examined at ENT clinic if TR patient.)
(Date of initial examination by audiology technician if DR patient.)

Audiological test results provided to specialist:

Audiogram: ☐ Yes   ☐ No

Other (specify):   1_____
                2_____
                3_____
                4_____

Write down any additional facts about this patient that you feel the specialist should be aware of:

Direct GP Referral Pilot Project

External Specialist Examination

Hospital _____

Patient name: _____

Findings of History and Examination

S = Significant factor prompting further investigation/intervention.
P = Present but not significant.

Comment   Comment

Right ear   Left ear

Comment	S	P		S	P	Comment
_____	☐ S	☐ P	Sudden Onset of Loss	☐ S	☐ P	_____
_____	☐ S	☐ P	Fluctuating Loss	☐ S	☐ P	_____
_____	☐ S	☐ P	Loss in one ear Only	☐ S	☐ P	_____
_____	☐ S	☐ P	Earache	☐ S	☐ P	_____
_____	☐ S	☐ P	Tinnitus	☐ S	☐ P	_____
_____	☐ S	☐ P	History of Discharge	☐ S	☐ P	_____
_____	☐ S	☐ P	Active Discharge	☐ S	☐ P	_____
_____	☐ S	☐ P	Diseased Canal	☐ S	☐ P	_____
_____	☐ S	☐ P	Perforation	☐ S	☐ P	_____
_____	☐ S	☐ P	Inflamed Drum	☐ S	☐ P	_____
_____	☐ S	☐ P	Scarred/Atropic Drum	☐ S	☐ P	_____

Vertigo _____ ☐ S   ☐ P _____

Findings of Audiometry

☐ Significant Asymmetric Loss   ☐ Significant Conductive Loss

---

Other factors prompting further investigation/intervention

Action

Tick all that apply

☐ Degree of loss does not warrant Hearing Aid

☐ Appropriate to fit Hearing Aid

☐ Further Investigation required (ENSURE FACTORS ARE TICKED 'S' OR WRITTEN ABOVE)

☐ Medical Intervention required (ENSURE FACTORS ARE TICKED 'S' OR WRITTEN ABOVE)

☐ Review patient's ears again at later date

   (give reasons_____)

☐ Other_____

Examination blind to patient's route of referral   ☐ Yes   ☐ No

Should this patient have been referred to an ENT surgeon?   ☐ Yes   ☐ No

---

What form would this investigation take (Tick all that apply):

☐ More detailed examination

☐ Opinion of another specialist

☐ Additional testing

☐ Other_____

If additional testing is needed, specify what tests:

1 _____   4 _____

2 _____   5 _____

3 _____   6 _____

Only complete this section if a medical condition has been identified

If a medical condition has been identified for which the patient is (apparently) *not* receiving treatment please specify (do not include age-related hearing loss)

_____

Is this condition treatable or not?

☐ Yes   ☐ No   ☐ Cannot tell without further tests/examination

Given the age, health, etc of this patient and the type of treatment involved, would you recommend that the condition be treated?

☐ Yes   ☐ No   ☐ Cannot tell without further tests/examination

If treatable, how serious could the consequences be for this patient if this condition was not treated?

In near future:	☐ Not Serious	☐ Serious	☐ Very Serious	☐ Cannot tell
In long term:	☐ Not Serious	☐ Serious	☐ Very Serious	☐ Cannot tell

In your opinion, could this condition have developed in the time since the patient was last examined?

☐ Definitely	☐ Probably	☐ Could	☐ Probably	☐ Definitely
did	did	have	did not	did not

Any Additional Comments

_____

_____

_____

Appendix I.III

TTSA guidelines for technicians seeing DR patients

Liaison Group for Technicians, Therapists and Scientists in Audiology

Suggested criteria which should be satisfied before a patient referred directly to an Audiology Department by a G.P. may be fitted with a Hearing Aid.

1. The patient must be aged 60 or over.

2. The patient must have been seen by the G.P. and have had both ears dewaxed as necessary.

3. Directly referred patients may be seen by any qualified Audiology technician or Scientist for their audiometry. The taking of the history, the examination of the ears and the judgement of suitability for hearing aids, must be done by the Technicians of Senior Grade or above, or by Audiological Scientists of post-probationary grades (i.e. following successful completion of the Certificate of Audiological Competence).

4. This Direct Referral service shall apply only for patients referred for consideration for hearing aids. No other type of E.N.T. or hearing abnormality referral may be accepted directly from a G.P.

5. The Technician or Scientist may not proceed with the supply of any hearing aid system, without E.N.T. medical advice if any of the following conditions apply:
    a) Excessive wax in either ear.
    b) A perforated ear drum, an active discharge or a history of discharge from either ear.
    c) Otalgia affecting either ear.
    d) Vertigo. (As classically described - 'An hallucination of movement'. Not to be confused with the common unsteadiness of old age).
    e) Hearing loss of sudden onset.
    f) Sudden deterioration in an existing hearing loss.
    g) Hearing loss subject to fluctuation beyond that associated with colds.
    h) Hearing loss where audiometry shows an average air/bone gap in excess of 30 dB in either ear. (The B/C audiometry, masked as necessary, should be tested from at least 500Hz to 2000Hz).
    i) Asymmetrical hearing losses: as an index of suspicion a difference between ears in BO thresholds of 20 dB or greater at .5, 1, 2 or 4 KHz may be used.
    j) Any other unusual presenting features at the discretion of the Audiology Technician or Audiological Scientist.

Revised 9.1.89

Calculations used in the comparison of a mixture of DR and TR systems with TR on its own

1. The computations below were done separately for each expert assessor. For brevity, detailed calculations are presented for the first expert only.

2. *Estimation of the Proportion of Patients with Potentially Serious Conditions that come through DR.*
   4.2% of DR patients had potentially serious conditions, compared to 8.1% of TR patients. Also, during the last part of the pilots around 36% of all hearing aid patients were DRs, and 64% TRs (see chapter 21). Therefore out of every 100 patients, on average 36 will be DRs with 36 * 0.42 = 1.51 potentially serious, and 64 will be TRs with 64 * 0.81 = 5.16 potentially serious. The expected total number of potentially serious cases per 100 patients is therefore 1.51 + 5.16 = 6.67, of which 1.51, or 23%, come through the DR system, and the other 77% through the TR system.

3. The same calculations for expert 2 indicate that the overall number of potentially serious cases per 100 patients is 9.24, with 2.27 or 25% coming through DR.

4. *Computation of 95% confidence interval on success rate for DR and TR combined.*
   The confidence interval is computed for a fixed value for the proportion of potentially serious cases coming through DR of 23% (see above).

Let
   T = proportion of DR patients with potentially serious pathology cross referred by technicians.
   D = proportion of patients with potentially serious pathology correctly managed by ENT doctors.

Assuming that T and D are each binomially distributed variables, we have, on the basis of the first expert's assessments:

Expectation(T) = $t = 5 / 10$		= 0.5
Variance(T) = $t * (1 - t)) / N = 0.5 * 0.5 / 10$		= 0.025
Expectation(D) = $d = 8 / 14$		= 0.41
Variance(D) = $0.41 * 0.59 / 14$		= 0.01423

Now,
   Expectation(potentially serious cases detected under DR) = $E(DR) = t * d$
   Expectation(potentially serious cases detected under TR) = $E(TR) = d$

Therefore, under the assumption that 23% of serious cases come through DR:
   Expectation(potentially serious cases detected under DR and TR combined)
   = E(DR/TR mixed) = $E(DR) * 0.23 + E(TR) * 0.77$
   $= t * d * 0.23 + d * 0.77$
   $= 0.363$ (or 36.3%)

The difference between the systems can be expressed as
   Difference $= D - T * D * 0.23 - D * 0.77$
   $= D * 0.23 * (1 - T)$

With

Expectation(Difference) = d * 0.23 * (1 - t) = 0.0472 (or 4.7%)

Also,

Variance(Difference) = V(D * 0.23 * (1 - T))

This is of the form V(XY), where X = D * 0.23, and Y = 1 - T. Assuming X and Y are independent variables,

V(XY) = V(X) * V(Y) + E(Y) * E(Y) * V(X) + E(X) * E(X) * V(Y)

We have

E(D * 0.23) = 0.41 * 0.23   = 0.0943
V(D * 0.23) = 0.23 * 0.23 * V(D) = 0.000753
E(1 - T) = 1 - 0.5   = 0.5
V(1 - T) = V(T)   = 0.025

So,

V(Diff) = 0.000753 * 0.025 + 0.5 * 0.5 * 0.000753 + 0.0943 * 0.0943
          * 0.025
        = 0.000429

Standard deviation(Diff) = 0.021 (or 2.1%)

Taking plus and minus two standard deviations provides approximate 95% limits on the value of the difference. Therefore:

Expected difference between TR and a DR/TR mix   = 4.7%
Lower 95% confidence limit = 4.7 - 2 * 2.1   = 0.5%
Upper 95% confidence limit = 4.7 + 2 * 2.1   = 8.9%

Thus, under a mix of DR and TR systems (with 23% of all potentially serious cases coming through DR) the expectation is that 4.7% of potentially serious cases will be missed that would be picked up under TR alone, with a 95% confidence interval on this figure of 0.5% up to 8.9%.

It is important to note that these estimates are only true for the specific value of 23% of potentially serious cases coming through DR. If this proportion is higher, then the advantage of TR over the combination of systems improves.

5. The corresponding results for the second expert are an estimated difference between TR alone and DR/TR combined of 4.4%, with a 95% confidence interval of 0.8% up to 8.0%.

6. *Rates of Potentially Serious Failures over all Patients.*
    It was estimated in (2) above that 6.7% of all patients (DR and TR together, first expert) attend with potentially serious conditions. The success of doctors with potentially serious cases was 41%, therefore we expect 6.7 * (1 - 0.41) = 3.95% of all patients to be potentially serious fails if all patients came through TR. The success rate of the DR/TR mix was estimated as 36%, indicating that under this arrangement 6.7 * (1 - 0.36) = 4.29% of all patients would have potentially serious conditions that are not detected.

Appendix I.V

Methodological and technical details of the cost analysis

Appendix I.V.I: Factors with cost implications not included in the analysis

Appendix I.V.II: Details of time and cost estimates

Appendix I.V.III: Technical details of costing

I.V.I Factors with cost implications not included in the analysis

1. DEWAXING The assumption has been made that overall costs of dewaxing will be approximately the same for both systems. This is reasonable given that (in theory) a patient either needs dewaxing or doesn't, irrespective of the route they come through. The cost of wax removal is also assumed to be more-or-less the same whether a patient is dewaxed at the GP clinic or the hospital.

    At some Centres, a small number of DR patients who attend with wax are sent straight back to their GP for dewaxing. In comparison with TR - where ENT would normally dewax such patients - this probably results in a slight overall increase in cost due to wasted time at the Hearing Aid Centre.

2. NUMBER OF APPOINTMENT. The cost analysis assumes that all TR and DR patients have three appointments at the hospital/Centre: first appointment (for examination, testing and impressions), fitting, and follow-up - with the exception of cross-referred DRs who have an additional appointment for an ENT examination. In practice, however, a proportion of both types have extra appointments (e.g. if the impressions have to be done on a different day). In most Centres and for both groups the percentage was fairly small. In only two Centres, Red and Grey, was the percentage of patients having an extra appointment large enough to affect the overall costings by more than £1. At both of these Centres this factor relates to TR patients only, and increases the average service cost to these patients by roughly £1.50. We have computed that, on the average, the additional cost incurred due to an extra appointment - assuming that it is for ear impressions or testing which could not be done at the first appointment - is a little under £2.

3. USHERING OF PATIENTS. Under TR, at the first appointment, patients are seen separately by a technician and an ENT doctor. In some places the Hearing Aid Centre and ENT department are housed apart, and patients need to be ushered from one to the other, in some cases more than once. A good proportion of hearing aid patients are disabled, which adds to this problem. Also, this system can involve repetition of information from the patient to the various staff. The great majority of DR patients are seen by a single individual who conducts all of the procedures in one go in one place. There are clearly time and cost savings here, but of an unknown quantity.

4. STATIONARY AND STAMPAGE. These have not been costed because the costs are generally met by the hospital rather than the departments themselves. However, it is worth noting that, insofar as they are related to the number of appointments a patients has, there is likely to be a small overall extra cost associated with DR, due to cross-referred patients.

I.V.II Details of time and cost estimates

1. GP CLINIC TIME. For TR patients, 5 minutes of GP clinic time has been allocated. The interviews with TR patients suggested that this

would be an appropriate figure. The basis upon which GP Clinic time is costed includes not only the salary of the GP themselves, but also the costs of clerical and support staff, and materials and medicines (see appendix I.V.III, point 1). Therefore the figure of 5 minutes also allows for 5 minutes of clerical time, plus material costs.

It is difficult to say whether DR patients consume any more GP resources than TR patients. During the pilot projects the great majority of GPs directly referred no more than 2 or 3 patients, and so it is impossible to obtain an accurate answer to this, even from GPs themselves. Given that GPs should, theoretically, be a bit more thorough with DR patients to ensure that they match the referral criteria, costings have been computed using two different figures: 5 minutes (i.e. the same as TR) and 7 minutes.

2. TIMES SPENT BY TECHNICIANS ON AUDIO TESTING, IMPRESSIONS, AND FITTING. At each Centre, technicians recorded the times they spent on these procedures for each DR patient they saw. Mean times were computed for each Centre, and the time given in figure 15.1 (in chapter 15) for each of these procedures is the mean of these means.

    The assumption is made that the amount of time spent is also the same for TR patients. However, the grades of technicians seeing DR and TR patients were not the same for both systems, and therefore the costings for these procedures differ between systems.

3. TIME SPENT BY TECHNICIANS ON HISTORY AND EAR EXAMINATION. As above, the time given in figure 15.1 is the 'mean of means' across all Centres. There were a few instances where technicians misunderstood what they were being asked to do, and instead of recording the time spent on the history and ear-examination, recorded the time for all of the procedures undertaken. In some cases, it was easy to subtract the times for other procedures to arrive at the correct figure. Where this was not possible, the data for the technician involved was excluded, and replaced with the overall mean for that Centre. For two Centres, Brown and Silver, it was necessary to exclude all of these timings, and substitute the overall mean across all of the other Centres.

4. TIME SPENT BY ENT DOCTORS ON ENT EXAMINATION. ENT doctors recorded the times that they spent with each DR patient at the safety-check examination, and this data has been used to estimate the times spent on ENT examinations of TR patients. There are good reasons for believing however, that this time - the mean of means is 7.1 minutes - underestimates that usually spent with traditionally referred patients. Firstly, prior to the DR schemes a number of ENT doctors across the twelve centres (38 in all) were asked how long, on average, they spent with TR patients. The mean of the responses was 11.3 minutes; but several said that it would be a few minutes less for straight-forward hearing aid cases. Secondly, when they were interviewed towards the end

of the pilot schemes, ENT doctors were asked about how the time spent on a safety-check compared with a normal ENT examination. Out of a total of 21 doctors, 9 said the times were about the same, and 12 that they spent less time over a safety-check. Estimates of how much less ranged from 3 mins to 10 mins, with a median of 5 minutes.

On the basis of the above, costings have been derived using two values for the ENT examination time. The first being the time spent on safety-checks, which we can be confident represents a lower bound on the actual time, and the second being this figure plus 4 minutes, which gives a reasonable upper bound. This latter figure (mean 11.1 minutes) is almost identical to the mean of the doctors' estimates for the time spent with TR patients, and co-incidently is also almost identical to the mean time that technicians spend on the history and examination of DR patients(11.2 minutes).

5. TIME SPENT BY ENT DOCTORS ON PAPERWORK. Although this item may look trivial, in fact in some cases doctors spend longer on the paperwork than with the patient themselves. The principal element of the paperwork for doctors is writing back to the referring GP. Having asked a couple of senior registrars about this, an average time of 3 minutes paperwork per patient has been allocated.

6. TIMES SPENT BY TECHNICIANS ON PAPERWORK. An average time of 5 minutes at each appointment has been allocated here. This seems a reasonable overall average, from discussions with some of the technicians involved. It is also the figure that Brooks (1991) used. For the first appointment with DR patients, however, the time has been increased to 8 minutes, to allow for the technician taking over the ENT doctor's job of replying to the GP, or cross-referring to ENT if necessary.

7. TIMES SPENT BY CLERICAL OFFICERS. An average of 15 minutes clerical officer work per patient appointment has been used, increased to 20 minutes for the first appointment (for TR patients this is 15 minutes ENT clerical and 5 minutes Audiology clerical, for DRs it is 20 minutes Audiology clerical). The tasks covered by this time include: sending appointments out, rearranging appointments, registering patients, making out files and updating files, recalling hospital notes, typing letters, arranging hospital transport where necessary. The total amount of clerical work has been assumed to be the same for both DR and TR, and therefore the actual times used are not critical to the cost comparison of the systems.

8. TIME SPENT BY ENT DOCTORS WITH CROSS-REFERRED DR PATIENTS. The time given here is the mean of means based on the actual times spent with these patients during the pilots.

9. COST OF HEARING AID. There was no evidence that the types of aid fitted differed greatly between the DR and TR systems, and therefore a fixed price per fitting was adopted. There are slight variations in price

between different BE series aids, and so a weighted average was used based on a mix of 90% series 10 aids and 10% series 30 aids, which is roughly the overall mix found in practice. The cost includes VAT.

10. COST OF EAR-MOULD. The cost here is that reported by Brooks (1990), plus 6% to update the figure to 1991.

11. COST OF ACCESSORIES. The accessories to the aid itself include a storage box, batteries, and relevant literature. As above, the figure given by Brooks (1990) has been used, incremented by 6%.

12. INSTRUMENTATION. During the process of provision a variety of instrumentation may be used. The principal ones are an audiometer, an otoscope, impression syringe, and earlight. Also numerous other items may be required, such as tuning forks, pliers, tweezers, tools for modifying the earmould, a tape recorder, and so on. Brooks determined a cost of 30 pence per fitting for instrumentation, based on an eight-year life-span and 800 fittings per year. This does not include ENT instrumentation, which is probably at least as much again given that most of these items will be duplicated in ENT, and they may utilize other, more specialized, equipment.

Fortunately the costs involved here are small, and not critical to the comparison of systems. Accordingly, we have allocated an instrumentation cost of 10 pence per appointment in Audiology (which over three appointments equals Brooks' figure of 30p), plus another 10 pence for each ENT appointment (i.e. TR patients and DR cross-referrals).

I.V.III Technical details of costing

1. COST OF GP CLINIC TIME. To compute these costs, figures provided by the Department of Health were used. These include an estimate of £7.79 per GP consultation in 1990/91, which was incremented by 6% to give £8.26 for 1991/92. The average length of a consultation was 9.3 minutes, making an average rate of £0.89 per minute. This covers all clinic costs, including clerical help and materials.

2. PROCEDURES ON DR PATIENTS UNDERTAKEN BY TECHNICIANS. The cost of each of these procedures is based upon the actual times recorded by technicians. The following measures were computed separately for each procedure at each centre: a) the mean time spent by each grade of technician on the procedure, as a fraction of an hour; b) rate of pay per hour for that grade (based on the mid-point of the scale - except where it was known that the technicians were at the top of MTO2 - including superannuation etc, allowing for 10 days public holidays, 4 or 5 weeks leave (depending on grade) and 1 week sick leave); c) the percentage of patients seen by that grade. The cost per patient for each procedure was then computed by multiplying these together and summing over all grades involved. This method gives estimates equivalent to computing a separate cost for each patient (based on the grade of technician and time taken) and taking the mean over all patients.

The same approach - of computing times, pay-rates, and percentages of patients seen, separately for each grade - was applied to every element in the costing exercise that involved either technicians or doctors. This yields the most accurate estimates of cost, and also preserves maximum variability.

3. PROCEDURES ON TR PATIENTS UNDERTAKEN BY TECH-NICIANS. The data collected on samples of TR patients prior to DR yielded figures for the percentages of patients seen by each grade of technician, at each Centre. Times spent with these patients were not available, however. Therefore the times spent with DR patients were used. Where there was a grade of technician seeing TR patients for which no time estimate was available (i.e. no technician of this grade saw DR patients), the mean time for all technicians at that centre was substituted.

4. COST OF ENT EXAMINATION OF CROSS-REFERRED DR PATIENTS. From the forms completed by ENT doctors, the actual grades of doctors involved and the times they took were known. Rates of pay were based on the mid-point of each grade scale.

5. COST OF ENT EXAMINATION OF TR PATIENTS. From the samples of TR patients fitted before DR, the percentages of patients examined by each grade of doctor were available. High and low estimates of the mean time taken by each grade were derived from the safety-checks of DR patients, as explained in appendix I.V.II. Where a grade of doctor was involved with TR patients for which a time estimate was not available (i.e. no doctor of this grade had seen DR patients), the mean time across all doctors at that centre was used. In addition, there were two or three instances where the mean time for a grade was based on very few cases and did not look at all representative: overall means were also substituted for these. For example, at one centre a doctor who examined a high proportion of TR patients had seen just one DR, and spent 25 minutes with them. We considered it inappropriate to apply this extreme figure to all of the TR patients they had seen.

6. COST OF TIMES SPENT BY TECHNICIANS AND DOCTORS ON PAPERWORK. As with the preceding procedures, these costs for both DR and TR take into account the grades and percentages of patients seen by each.

7. COST OF CLERICAL OFFICER TIME. No information was available on the grades of clerical officer employed at each centre, therefore all clerical work was costed at the same rate, which was the mid-point of scale 2, equal to £4.50 per hour.

162

Appendix I.VI

Comments by Mr Charles Smith

Comments by Mr Charles Smith

Dear David,

It was kind of you and your colleagues to invite me to make a personal comment on our attempt to evaluate the pros and cons of direct referral of patients with hearing problems to Audiology Departments.

As you will learn from my findings at the four centres that I have visited, there is very little risk, in my opinion, of missing serious pathology as a result of a Direct Referral scheme. However, I believe a dogmatic statement to the effect that Direct Referral is the ideal solution for the hearing impaired, even if this is only for the over 65s, would not be in the interests of the Deaf. It would oversimplify and minimize the problem of fitting hearing aids satisfactorily. I would want to emphasize that successful fitting may require a team effort sometimes involving Consultant Otologist, Audiological Scientist, Senior Audiological Technician and possibly Voluntary Visitor for the Deaf. As you probably know the British Association of the Hard of Hearing has gone as far as publishing a protocol for Voluntary Visitors because of the unsatisfactory outcome when patients are fitted with hearing aids in the National Health Service under the present scheme, and there is no reason to believe that Direct Referral would be any better.

Unfortunately one has to consider the political significance of reports within the National Health Service and any report which underestimated the difficulties of fitting hearing aids to people, especially those with neuro-sensory deafness,would reinforce the present tendency to underestimate the disability of deafness compared with other disabilities such as blindness. Furthermore there is no doubt in my mind that in the present state of knowledge it is more difficult to fit an aid satisfactorily than it is to correct a simple visual defect by prescribing spectacles. I do not need to remind you that although spectacles with ordinary magnifying lenses can be bought across the counter, the prescription of spectacles can only be carried out by fully qualified ophthalmic opticians with a University degree. I would hope that any report that we produced would emphasise the need to strive to improve the qualifications and training of all those involved with the management of people with hearing defects.

I think this is all I can usefully say without writing a thesis on 'The fitting of Hearing Aids to patients with Neuro-sensory Deafness'. Do let me know if you want me to enlarge on any of the topics that I have raised.

With Best Wishes.

Yours sincerely,

Charles W Smith

Appendix I.VII

Example form for use by GPs when referring

Direct Referral Scheme: GP Referral Form

NOTE: Do not use this form for hearing aid repairs. Repair clinics are held every Thursday afternoon at the Hearing Aid Centre; no appointment necessary.

Patient name:

Address:

Telephone:

Date of birth: _ (note: Patients Must be *at Least 60 Years Old*)

First-time referral / reassessment (please delete as appropriate)

To be suitable for Direct Referral, all boxes below must be ticked

No excessive wax in either ear* ☐

No active discharge or history of discharge ☐

No skin disease in ear canals ☐

No perforated or inflamed ear drums ☐

No earache ☐

No tinnitus (other than occasional/transient) ☐

No sudden onset of loss or sudden deterioration of loss ☐

No fluctuating loss (beyond that associated with colds) ☐

No markedly asymmetrical hearing loss ☐

No vertigo (not the common unsteadiness of old age) ☐

* The patient's ears must be clear of wax before referring

Signed_____ Date _____

Other comments:

GP name and address:

Please return this form to: Hearing Aid Centre (Direct Referral)
Somewhere Hospital
Sometown
Someshire   tel 111-111-1111

Part II

Survey of Pre-existing Direct Referral Systems in England

Linda Mason
David Reeves
Helen Prosser
Chris Kiernan

24 Introduction

24.1 Aims of the survey

24.1.1 A survey of all NHS Hearing Aid Centres in England was conducted in February to April 1991. The aim of the survey was to assess the extent to which Direct Referral procedures for hearing aid provision (defined in Part I, section 1.2) have been set up under local initiatives in the National Health Service. This information was then used as a basis for selecting a sample of Centres to be visited with a view to gathering detailed information on the organization and operation of the schemes, and on the problems and benefits experienced.

25 Results of the Postal Survey

25.1 Methodology

25.1.1 The survey was conducted in two stages, the first of which involved sending a postal questionnaire to all Hearing Aid Centres in England with a covering letter explaining the purpose of the survey. A reminder was sent one month later to Centres that had not returned the questionnaire. Any not responding to the reminder were telephoned and the details requested over the phone.

25.1.2 In order to promote a high response rate the questionnaire was kept short and concise. The main priority was to obtain a clear picture of the extent of Direct Referral throughout the country. Some additional questions for those who had operated or were operating DR were included. This was to enable a selection to be made of Centres from whom more detailed information on Direct Referral would be obtained. The survey questionnaire appears in appendix II. I.

25.2 Results

25.2.1 *Number of DR Schemes.*
158 questionnaires were sent, of which 144 were returned. (91% response rate). Of these, 56 (39%) currently operated or had operated Direct Referral. This figure includes 1 scheme suspended at the time of the survey whilst a further 3 had been suspended some time in the past, but had later been reinstated. Two other Centres had completely halted DR for the foreseeable future.

25.2.2 *Regional Distribution* (table 25.1).
The majority of DR schemes have been set up in the South East of England, mainly throughout the Thames region. Indeed, the four Thames RHA's between them account for fully 50% of all schemes in existence. A smaller concentration is located in the North-West of the country.

25.2.3 *Starting Date* (table 25.2).
The longest known time that Direct Referral has been in operation at any Centre is since 1972, and this is since the hospital concerned first opened. The majority of DR systems were set up during the late 1980's and early 1990's. In particular, a large number (16) started operating in 1990.

Table 25.1
Regional distribution of DR schemes

Regional Health Authority	No. of Direct Referral schemes
North West Thames	11
South East Thames	8
North East Thames	6
North West Region	6
Yorkshire	6
Mersey	5
South West Thames	3
South West Region	3
Wessex	3
Oxford	2
Northern	2
East Anglia	1
Trent	0
West Midlands	0
Total	56

Table 25.2
Starting date of Direct Referral schemes

Starting date	No. of schemes
1972	1
1975	1
1976	2
1977	1
1978	1
1980	5
1981	2
1983	2
1985	3
1986	3
1987	3
1988	6
1989	3
1990	16
1991 (up to April)	2

(Starting dates were not known for 5 centres)

26 Selection of Centres for Interviewing

26.1 Selection criteria

26.1.1 A total of twenty one Centres were chosen for interviewing. Selection was based upon a wide range of criteria. The decision was taken not to attempt to draw up a 'representative' sample, but instead to select Centres on the basis of trying to maximise the variety of experience and type of scheme. It was felt that this approach would be the most fruitful in terms of the information produced.

26.1.2 Important characteristics of the 21 Centres are given in table 26.1. To maintain confidentiality Centres are referred to by number and not by name. The criteria used for selecting the sample were as follows:

1) ABANDONMENT OF A DIRECT REFERRAL SYSTEM
   All Centres that had operated Direct Referral but then stopped were interviewed in order to ascertain the reasons for stoppage. A total of six were included, although three of these had since restarted and one other had definite plans to restart as soon as certain problems were resolved.

2) LENGTH OF TIME DIRECT REFERRAL HAD BEEN OPERATING
   A broad range of Direct Referral life-span was sought. A number of Centres were chosen on the basis that DR had been running for a long time (i.e. 10 years or more). It was expected that these Centres would have resolved any problems and the scheme would be running smoothly. It was hoped that insight could be gained from these as to how problems which had occurred had been overcome. In contrast to these were Centres that started DR within the last few years. The reason for inclusion being that staff responsible for setting up the scheme would be available for interview, and they would have first-hand knowledge about the reasons for introducing DR and the early progress of their scheme. However, no schemes which started after mid-1990 were chosen because it was felt that these had not been running for long enough.

3) MAIN SITE VERSUS COMMUNITY PROVISION
   Inclusion was also based on the variety of sites at which directly referred patients are seen. This includes schemes at both main hospitals and those at peripheral hospitals or clinics.

4) NUMBER OF PATIENTS SEEN UNDER DIRECT REFERRAL
   The numbers of patients seen under Direct Referral was another selection factor. Again a wide range was deemed important, as the size and extent of the schemes may influence the types of problems encountered. The average number of DR patients seen per month varied from a minimum of 22 at one Centre up to a maximum of 150 at another.

Table 26.1
Direct Referral schemes
chosen for interview

Place	DRs per month	Site	Start date	Special features
Schemes continuous since inception				
1	35	M+P	'88	
2	90	M+P	'84	GPs refer any patient with hearing difficulty
3	35	M	'76	
4	90	M+P	'88	
5	80	M+P	'80	
7	22	M	'87	50% Cross-referral rate
9	45	M+P	'88	No age limit
11	140	M	'89	Has been evaluated internally
12	50	M	'90	Pilot study done
13	30	M	'72	
14	50	M	'89	
16	30	M+P	'80	
18	120	M+P	'90	Problems with staff shortages
20	40	M	'88	
21	150	M+P	'78	
Schemes that are / have been suspended				
10	50	M+P	'90	Lack of money + staff shortage
15	50	M	'90	Staffing difficulties on previous scheme
17	25	M+P	'90	Previous scheme suspended
19	50	M+P	'80	Staff shortages
Schemes that have stopped				
6	–	M	'86	Waiting list for DR longer than for ENT. Stopped '87
8	–	–	DK	Problems with GP referrals. Stopped '86

Site: M = Main site P = Peripheral site

5) GEOGRAPHICAL SPREAD

Further selection was based on locality. A wide geographical spread was aimed at, so as to include sites under the direction of different health authorities, and also both rural and urban areas where problems – such as patient access – may differ.

6) STATEMENTS OF EXPERIENCE

A number of Centres volunteered comments about their system. Some Centres were selected on the basis of the comments made. For example, one Centre was selected because they operate an unusual system whereby GPs refer all patients with hearing difficulty to the audiological technicians.

26.1.3 Staffing level is another important factor along which Centres differ. However, information on this was not available prior to selection. Instead,

Table 26.2
Audiological staff employed whilst Direct Referral is/was in operation

Centre	Audiological Scientist		TECHNICIANS		
		Senior	Junior+student		Total
1	0 (0)	3 (1)	0 (1)		3
2	0 (0)	4 (1)	1 (2)		5
3	0 (#)	2 (#)	1 (#)		3
4	0 (0)	6 (0)	5 (0)		11
5	0 (#)	3 (#)	6 (#)		9
6	0 (#)	3 (#)	2 (#)		5
7	0 (0)	3 (0)	0 (0)		3
8	0 (0)	2 (0)	0 (0)		2
9	1 (0)	2 (0)	5 (0)		8
10	0 (0)	2 (0)	1 (2)		3
11	0 (0)	3 (0)	5 (0)		8
12	2 (1)	5 (0)	6 (0)		13
13	2 (1)	3 (0)	1 (2)		6
14	1 (1)	2 (0)	2 (0)		5
15	0 (0)	4 (1)	3 (0)		7
16	3 (0)	6 (0)	5 (0)		14
17	0 (0)	4 (0)	0 (0)		4
18	0 (0)	2 (0)	3 (0)		5
19	1 (0)	4 (0)	2 (0)		7
20	1 (0)	2 (2)	0 (3)		3
21	0 (0)	7 (1)	9 (0)		16

Note: Figures in brackets are numbers of vacancies
= Not known

Table 26.3
ENT consultants and audiological physicians employed whilst Direct Referral is/was in operation

Centre	ENT Consultants	Audiological Physicians	Total
1	2	0	2
2	3	1	4
3	2	#	#
4	#	1	#
5	2	#	#
6	#	#	#
7	2	0	2
8	3	0	3
9	#	#	#
10	#	#	#
11	4	0	4
12	4	0	4
13	3	0	3
14	#	#	#
15	#	#	#
16	5	1	6
17	2	0	2
18	3	0	3
19	2	0	2
20	2	1	3
21	4	1	5

= Not known

details on staffing were collected at the interviews subsequent to selection. This data appears in tables 26.2 and 26.3. It show a good range of staffing levels within the selected sample; with the number of audiological staff (scientists and technicians) varying between a low of just 2 and a high of 16; and ENT consultants (plus audiological physicians) ranging between 2 and 6.

26.2 Number of staff interviewed

26.2.1 The aim was to conduct interviews in each Centre with both the head technician and a consultant with good knowledge of the DR scheme. Whilst there was no difficulty in arranging interviews with all 21 head technicians, in 9 Centres it was not possible to talk with a consultant. At four of these however, the consultant instead completed a questionnaire based on the interview schedule and returned it. This makes a total number of returns from consultants of 16. Copies of the interview schedules appear in appendix II.II.

27 Reasons Given for the Introduction of Direct Referral

27.1 The reasons given
(tables 27.1, 27.2)

27.1.1 The question 'What were the reasons behind the introduction of Direct Referral?' was asked of both technicians and consultants. Even when the interviewee was not in employment at the Centre at the start of the scheme, most were able to suggest the reasons as to why DR was introduced. In some cases however, technicians and consultants from the same Centre gave different reasons.

Table 27.1
Reasons given by technicians for the introduction of Direct Referral

Reason	Number	Percentage
A) Long waiting list for ENT	11	52%
B) To eliminate the wait for those that do not need to see the ENT consultant	6	29
C) Hearing aid patients were being put back on the waiting list as they were not urgent	1	5
D) To bring more work into the hearing aid dept	2	10
E) Job satisfaction for technicians	1	5
F) To give the hearing aid dept control over the number of patients coming through from ENT per session	1	5
G) To free ENT clinics for more serious cases	2	10
H) To speed up the ENT clinics	1	5
I) To see if patients respond more readily to an aid issued through Audiology only	1	5
J) Quality assurance	2	10

NB - More than one response may have been given, so %'s add to more than 100%

27.1.2 Both technicians and consultants gave the main reasons for their Centre introducing Direct Referral as being: a) the long waiting list for ENT (given by 52% of technicians and 44% of consultants); and b) to eliminate the wait for those patients who don't need to see a doctor (29% and 31% respectively).

27.1.3 Although both answers are similar, showing concern for the length of wait, those answers that were classified under b) specifically mentioned that there is no need for a straightforward hearing aid patient to be seen in ENT:

Table 27.2
Reasons given by consultants for the introduction of Direct Referral

Reason	Number	Percentage
To eliminate the wait for those patients who do not need to see a doctor	7	44%
Long waiting list for ENT	5	31
To free ENT clinics for more serious cases	5	31
Hearing aid patients were being pushed back on the waiting list because they are not urgent cases	1	6
To speed up the ENT clinics	1	6
The technicians can take as good an examination and history as the doctors	1	6
To evaluate Direct Referral to see if it is safe	1	6

NB - More than one response may have been given, so %'s add to more than 100%

'It's just a waste of resources – in my view – people with just a hearing problem to be seen by a consultant it's just a waste of money, resources, time everything that is valuable is wasted by doing it that way and it's only historic after all, you just have to break some of these historic links. I was really aggrieved about the waste of resources, it was just a total utter waste of ENT time' (technician).

'It seemed to the most part inappropriate for a patient who was elderly and has a very high probability of age induced deafness going through the process of seeing a consultant surgeon when all they need is a hearing aid' (consultant).

'Mr X (consultant) is the one who wanted to do this because his list was growing rapidly and the waiting times were becoming too long and he said 'well really it's a waste of my time seeing a lot of these people, they don't need to see me at all, they need to see you' (technician).

27.1.4 Concern was also expressed over the length of wait in the ENT clinic itself:

'Also just the fact that people would maybe be waiting a couple of hours in clinics for a 3 minute consultation' (technician).

27.1.5 A couple of technicians pointed out that patients would be examined by junior ENT doctors rather than by a consultant. They felt this had little value for the patient:

'They would be seen by, as I say, very junior doctors who really weren't contributing a great deal'.

'Essentially what was happening is that the majority of patients obviously were elderly and they were getting to see a junior doctor in the ENT who knew very little about them. They came along, he did a history and they said 'I've been deaf for the last 15 years, like to try a hearing aid' and he says 'ah you're deaf'. They said 'that's why we came' – so it's a waste of time'.

27.1.6 As well as being introduced in order to benefit straightforward hearing aid patients, DR is also established so as to relieve ENT staff by freeing clinics and cutting waiting lists. This enables the more serious cases to be seen earlier. A greater proportion of consultants (31%) suggested this as a reason for introducing DR than technicians (10%):

'Secondly we wanted to free medical staff time to see those patients who really did need to see them thus making the medical clinics more efficient in that they were uncluttered with simple hearing aid cases' (consultant).

27.1.7 The remaining reasons were mentioned by only the occasional technician or consultant. One consultant believed that as the technicians could take as good an examination and history as the doctors there was no need for referral to ENT:

'There was so little time in the clinic for taking a decent history and so on that the technicians could just as well take just as good a history, just as good an examination as the doctors were giving the patients because the technicians are skilled' (consultant).

27.1.8 The aim of giving the Hearing Aid Centre control over the number of patients coming through per session was mentioned by one technician:

'It is better for technicians because they have got their booked patients instead of just having patients thrown at them from a clinic' (technician).

27.1.9 Introducing more work into the Hearing Aid Centre was the main reason for starting DR in two of the Centres, although the background to this differed somewhat:

'It was as far as I understand it, to get more work into the department because they had quite a few technicians here, but it's quite a small area that we cover' (technician).

'I worked for a consultant who believed that we didn't have that much work to do ... so in his infinite wisdom he decided to keep us busy because that's what we needed to be, we might as well just take the referrals from the GPs rather than going through his clinic' (technician)

27.1.10 Quality assurance was also given as a reason by a couple of technicians. It was felt that the benefits of DR would improve the quality of service to the patients and their families.

28 DR Schemes that have Stopped

28.1 Reasons for stopping
(tables 28.1, 28.2, 28.3)

28.1.1 Of the 144 Hearing Aid Centres that replied to the postal questionnaire only six acknowledged that any stoppage or suspension of DR had taken place. Of the six, three had been suspended in the past but Direct Referral reintroduced after steps were taken to overcome the problems that had occurred. One is suspended for the present (i.e. at the time of the survey) whilst the remaining two have stopped for the foreseeable future. Interviews were conducted at all 6 of these Centres.

Table 28.1

Stoppage / suspension of Direct Referral (6 Schemes)

	Number
Suspended for the present	1
Suspended in past	3
Stopped for foreseeable future	2

Table 28.2

Reasons given for stoppage / suspension of Direct Referral (A total of six schemes included)

Reason	Number
Staff shortages	5
Too many patients needing dewax	2
The waiting list became longer for Direct Referral than for ENT	1
Too many inappropriate referrals (not counting patients with wax)	1
Increasing number of Direct Referrals including from out of the district	1

NB - more than one reason may have been given.

Table 28.3

Who took the decision to end /suspend the scheme

Person	Number
ENT consultant	2
Head of Audiology dept	2
Joint decision between ENT and Audiology	2

179

28.1.2 The major reason for stoppage/suspension in all Centres bar one, was staff shortages:

'Lack of technicians to actually do the work'.

'Lack of staff.'

'It was actually a problem with staffing.'

28.1.3 Staff leaving and not being replaced was a common problem:

'I lost X and Y went off, she was another student that I had that left last August and I was never allowed to replace her and Z was on maternity leave and that left myself and another student to run the entire district' (technician).

'We established about 6 posts, then they all left. It left myself, a part-time technician and one student. The staff just went so quickly that we just couldn't cope with the workload so we had to rearrange doing things and we had to actually stop doing the DR system' (technician).

28.1.4 Additional reasons given were of a similar nature, the resources available not being sufficient to cope with the demand. This has been a particular problem where the number of referrals from outside the district have been on the increase. In extreme cases the waiting list for DR has become longer than that for ENT:

'The waiting list for Direct Referral is absolutely horrendous and will be horrendous until they get us more staff and a better department' (technician).

28.1.5 Lack of staff resulting in a very long waiting list was the primary reason for the permanent abandonment of DR at one Centre.

28.1.6 In addition to the problem of resources, the other major reason for stoppage/suspension was a poor quality of referrals coming from GPs. GPs were criticized for referring patients with wax in their ears, and also for not adhering to the specified criteria for referral:

'That became, well it was a major problem because we had to have medical staff on hand to remove the wax and I think about 30% of the patients who came up needed to have wax removed so it did slow down the process considerably' (technician)

'GPs were abusing it both consciously and unconsciously, consciously they were shunting patients onto the DR scheme who they knew had cholesteatoma and other conditions because they knew that they would be picked up by the technician and taken over by the hand to the ENT surgeon...' (technician)

28.1.7 The second Centre to permanently halt DR did so principally because of GP misuse and abuse of the system. It is of interest to note that in none of the Centres where DR had stopped was the safety of the procedure given as a reason.

29 GP Involvement in Direct Referral

29.1 How GPs were made aware of the schemes
(table 29.1)

29.1.1 Ten of the Centres used a mailshot of all GPs to notify them of the scheme. Word of mouth was used as a means of communication by a further 4 Centres, whilst at 2 the Family Practitioner Committee was informed, who in turn notified GPs. At one of the Centres the consultant wrote only to selected GPs to inform them of the DR scheme:

> 'It wasn't totally open access, I actually wrote to a number of GP practices, the senior partners, people I knew and said 'look, we'll offer you this facility if you will agree to these criteria and you will abide by it'.

Table 29.1
How GPs were made aware of the Direct Referral scheme

	Number	Percentage
Mailshot to all GPS	10	48%
Word of mouth	4	19
Mail to those in a specific area	2	10
Through the family practitioner committee	2	10
Mail to a few that the consultant knew	1	5
The GPs have not been made aware of the scheme - ENT sort the letters	1	5
Don't know	1	5

29.1.2 One Centre sent a circular to GP practices within a specific geographical area. In another, patients were referred to ENT but examined in the Hearing Aid Centre by technicians. A letter was sent afterwards to the patient's GP informing them of what had occurred. From this GPs began automatically referring to the Hearing Aid Centre.

29.1.3 One of the Centres has not informed the GPs that patients are being screened by technicians. In this instance the GPs send referral letters to the ENT dept who in turn pass them straight on to the audiological technicians.

29.2 Training offered to GPs using Direct Referral
(table 29.2)

29.2.1 Both technicians and consultants were asked if any training or presentation was offered to GPs regarding the DR scheme. The great majority of Centres (14) had not made any arrangements for this. Two Centres included

Table 29.2
Was any training or presentation given to the GPs?

	Number	Percentage
Yes	3	14%
No	14	67
Don't know	4	19

the subject of DR within their annual ENT study day for GPs, whilst another gave a series of lectures to GPs at the start of the scheme. The Head Technician at this Centre was hoping to repeat these as:

'I think it's a good idea to remind them that we're here'.

29.2.2 Information was missing / not relevant for 4 of the Centres.

29.3 GP Referral criteria
(table 29.3)

29.3.1 Technicians and consultants were asked if they had provided GPs with criteria to help them select appropriate patients for DR. Ten Centres replied that GPs were given a set of criteria although it was not always particularly detailed:

'The letter just specified people over 60 who had no previous ear disease and no discharge, no wax'.

Often the criteria were in the form of a checklist on the referral slip.

Table 29.3
Were GPs provided with a set of criteria to follow when selecting patients for Direct Referral?

	Number	Percentage
Yes	10	48%
No	7	33
Don't know	3	14
Not applicable (GPs not aware of scheme)	1	5

29.3.2 Seven Centres had not set any criteria for GPs. One of these did however contact the GP in cases where a patient was incorrectly referred:

'We are quite lucky here that we can phone our GPs and say to them you've done it wrong'

29.3.3 Another, which again had close links with the GPs said:

'I'm very lucky with the GPs in this area because they all know what to do'

29.3.4 Information was missing / not relevant for four of the Centres.

29.4 The minimum age for Direct Referral patients
(table 29.4)

29.4.1 Two Centres stated that they had no minimum age criteria for directly referred patients. One said that they took 'everybody from babies upwards'. The second said they had 'minimum criteria' as opposed to a minimum age. It is unknown whether this refers to adults only or children as well.

Table 29.4
Minimum age for Direct Referral patients

Age criteria	Number	Percentage
No age limit	2	10%
18+	1	5
60+	10	48
65+	7	33
70+	1	5

29.4.2 One Centre took adults aged 18 and over. Ten Centres – the largest group – specified 60 as the minimum age, whilst at a further 7 it was age 65. One Centre only took patients of 70 or over. This limit was not one that has been formally set:

'A loose sort of precedence has been set by the ENT side which is about 70 or over comes direct down to us'.

29.4.3 At one of the Centres where 65 was the minimum age, the technician spoke of hoping to open it out to all patients aged over 18 but felt this would present a problem for ENT, in that junior doctors would be deprived of the opportunity to get some experience in seeing hearing aid patients:

'I think perhaps work is such here at the moment that ENT need the work of the hearing aid people because they are finding that perhaps the junior ENT staff now here are not going to get the referrals, so they are not going to have the experience of actually dealing with that side of it'.

It will be seen later that this potential drawback of the DR system is an issue of concern to many consultants.

29.5 DR patients referred with ear abnormalities

29.5.1 The question 'what happens if the technician discovers something abnormal about a directly referred patient's ear or pattern of loss?' was asked of the technicians (nb this does not include the problem of wax). Nineteen Centres refer patients straight on to the ENT department. At one Centre patients can decide themselves whether to be referred back to their GP or immediately to the ENT department:

'If the patient's preference is that they may want to go back to the GP and discuss it further with the GP who may wish to refer the patient – they have their own favourite consultants for various reasons - so we send a letter to the GP saying we recommend this patient has an ENT opinion, most of the patients are quite happy to have an ENT opinion here'.

29.5.2 The remaining Centre usually refers the patient back to the GP unless immediate treatment is necessary.

30 Involvement of Technicians

30.1 The grades of technicians who examine Direct Referral patients
(tables 30.1, 30.2)

30.1.1 Two questions were asked with regard to the grades of the technical staff that examine DR patients:

a. What grade are the staff involved in examining Direct Referrals?

b. Is there a minimum grade / no. of years experience for a technician to reach before being allowed to examine DR patients?

Table 30.1

Audiological staff involved in examining DR patients

Centre	Aud. Scientist	— MTO GRADE — 5	4	3	2	1	Total
1	1	–	–	–	–	–	1
2	1	–	1	2	–	–	4
3	–	–	1	1	1	–	3
4	–	1	1	4	–	–	6
5	–	1	–	2	3	2	8
6	–	–	2	1	–	–	3
7	–	–	1	2	–	–	3
8	#	#	#	#	–	–	2
9	1	–	1	1	–	–	3
10	–	–	1	1	–	–	2
11	–	1	–	2	4	–	7
12	1	1	1	1	–	–	4
13	2	–	1	1	1	1	6
14	1	–	1	1	–	–	3
15	–	1	1	1	–	–	3
16	–	1	2	3	1	–	7
17	–	–	1	4	–	–	5
18	–	–	1	–	–	–	1
19	–	–	1	3	–	–	4
20	–	–	1	–	–	–	1
21	#	1	1	2	2	–	#

= Unknown

30.1.2 Two out of the 21 Centres had technicians of grade MTO1 carrying out DR examinations. These were at the Centres where there was no minimum grade set. At a further four the lowest grade involved was MTO2. At 2 of these Centres MTO2 was suggested as the minimum grade set for examining directly referred patients. The other 2 Centres gave 'senior' (i.e. MTO3 and above) as the minimum – one however did say that exceptions would be allowed according to the technician involved. At the remaining 15 Centres

Table 30.2

Minimum grade /no. of years experience that technicians must reach before being allowed to examine Direct Referral patients

	Number	Percentage
Senior grade	12	57%
MTO3 with exceptions if the basic grade has enough experience or is competent	1	5
MTO3 with juniors under supervision	1	5
MTO2 minimum	2	10
No criteria	2	10
Missing information	3	14

all technicians examining directly referred patients were at least MTO3. However, because many of the Centres trained their staff from being students they are aware of their standard of work and what they are capable of. The question of setting a particular grade or number of years experience therefore had not always arisen. If new staff were to be taken on then a minimum grade would be set which in many instances might be higher than that currently in use.

30.1.3 A number of head technicians did feel they would be cautious about letting new staff examine DR patients even at senior level, until they were fully satisfied with the standard of their work:

'I think my newest senior has done about 7 or 8 years so they're very well experienced. If I was using somebody new as a senior I would have to see what their work was like, I would have to see how competent I felt they were because I think with Direct Referrals you have to show a high level of competence than if you're just relying on people coming through clinics because somebody has to take the responsibility'.

30.1.4 Of the two head technicians who said they had set no minimum grade, one had trained the technicians in the department herself but would have had reservations over someone new coming into the department:

'If that's a student who I've had from day one who's always been brought up with DR, has always seen the patient come through, they're a student which has always seen the way to do it, now if I got somebody else who'd been 12 months in somebody else's department I'd probably have reservations on them being able to do it. I know of my staff who can stand here and detect an abnormality and I know the quality of my staff'.

30.1.5 The other had senior staff to oversee junior staff doing DR and felt this was sufficient to overcome any problems that may occur.

30.1.6 Where the minimum grade suggested was higher than that of the technicians actually doing DR, this can be explained in part by the fact that the grades set by the health authority may not be totally relevant to the number of years experience or the quality of work the technician does. The technician may do work closer to that of a higher grade but the health authority may not be able or willing to employ them at a higher scale.

30.1.7 Overall, the majority of technicians interviewed did feel that once a technician has reached senior status they should have enough experience to examine directly referred patients:

'I would say under normal circumstances 3 years, that's possibly being a bit on the excessively cautious side, I certainly wouldn't have a student doing it because you know it's well out of the range of a student and I think it's also a lot to ask somebody who's newly qualified to take on.'

30.1.8 One exception to this occurred in a Centre where although seniors are allowed to carry out the DR examination and take the history, the decision over whether to refer the patient on to ENT is always taken by the head of department.

30.2 Training given to technicians prior to undertaking Direct Referral
(table 30.3)

30.2.1 Head technicians were asked 'is any special or additional training given to technicians who are going to be involved in examining DR patients?' Of the 21 Centres involved, only one gave any practical training, this was under the supervision of senior medical staff yet:

'I would suggest that there wasn't actually very much extra knowledge that was required, it was more a question of gaining necessary experience and modifying techniques as much as anything'.

Table 30.3
Additional training given to technicians who are going to be involved in examining directly referred patients

	Number	Percentage
No additional training	8	38%
The work of technicians new to Direct Referral is supervised/checked by a senior member of staff	4	19
Technicians new to Direct Referral sit in on clinics	3	14
Practical training session	1	5
Missing information	5	24

30.2.2 In four of the Centres, although no extra training is given, the work of any new staff undertaking DR is supervised and/or checked by a senior technician. In a further 3 Centres, staff new to Direct Referral would spend time sitting in on DR clinics.

30.2.3 Eight Centres gave no mention of any training or supervision of technicians new to DR. At these Centres it was generally felt that the usual training the technicians receive is of a sufficiently high standard:

'It's all just included in their basic training which is pretty good here'.

'No, I can't really see any need. Our technicians are trained to a very high standard and we use exactly the same standard for both (Traditional Referral and Direct Referral)'.

30.3 Consultant confidence in the technicians' work
(table 30.4)

30.3.1 Consultants were asked how confident they felt that technicians were referring on to them all patients who needed a medical opinion. Overall, there was a high degree of confidence in the technicians. Out of 15 consultants that were asked, 7 replied that they felt confident whilst a further 7 felt very confident. The remaining consultant felt unable to comment on the technicians work:

'Well that's something that I don't know, all I can say is that touch wood, we haven't had any patients who have gone through the system and referred back in a great hurry ....and that's the only way I can assess it'.

Table 30.4
Levels of consultant confidence that 'technicians are referring on to ENT all those patients that need to be seen by a doctor'

	Number	Percentage
Very confident	7	44%
Confident	7	44
Not confident	0	0
Don't know	1	6
Missing information	1	6

30.3.2 However, it is probable that in Centres where consultants are not confident about the technicians' abilities DR is not likely to be introduced. In this survey none of the Centres where Direct Referral was stopped/ suspended suggested that a lack of confidence in the technicians was one of the reasons for halting the scheme.

30.4 Evaluation of the performance of technicians

30.4.1 Despite expressing high levels of confidence in the technicians, 15 out of the 16 consultants interviewed said that no attempt had been made to formally evaluate their performance. One Centre, as part of a study to evaluate DR, assessed the accuracy of the technicians work by having a surgeon also examine a sample of DR patients. The results and recommendations for management of the patient were compared. Those patients that were 'failed' by the technicians and 'passed' by the surgeon were found to be 'diagnostic nuances or wax problems'. And in those cases where patients were 'passed' by the technician and 'failed' by the surgeon:

'It wasn't a question of what the technician was missing, it was a question of matter of judgement, minor problems related to say, conductive hearing loss, possible minor problem related to the medical management of tinnitus, that was that kind of thing that was cropping up'.

30.4.2 All in all, the consultant was very satisfied that the technicians were providing a sufficient safety screen. This study has in fact been published in the Journal of Laryngology and Otology (Hawthorne, Nunez, Clark, and Robertshaw 1991).

30.5 Technicians and dewaxing

30.5.1 In only two of the 21 Centres did technicians dewax patients. This was introduced in one of the Centres as a direct result of high numbers of patients attending with wax during a trial project. In this Centre the technicians were trained to remove wax under the responsibility of the consultant:

'Each of our technicians has a card to say that they have had to, under supervision, remove wax in ten patients to the satisfaction of the medical staff and then have their card signed up that this has been done appropriately and in a correct manner. And we've got this documentation which we could then prove in court that technician X has been formally and correctly trained in the technique' (technician).

30.5.2 Since the introduction of wax removal by technicians, patients being referred with wax are no longer a major problem.

30.5.3 Another of the Centres previously employed a technician that was trained to dewax. The technician has since left and no one has been trained to take her place. The technician was taught initially because of a problem with the number of referrals coming through the Direct Referral system with wax. However:

'Since we've got the GPs trained as it were, we don't really have a problem' (technician).

30.5.4 Another Centre employed a technician who had been trained to remove wax whilst working at another hospital, but who did not dewax at the present time. The technician concerned felt it should be left up to the GP and the practice nurses to remove wax:

'GPs are awful about wax, diabolical, just won't accept that it's a primary level responsibility' (technician).

30.6 Should technicians be trained to dewax?

(table 30.5)

30.6.1 Both technicians and consultants were asked whether they thought technicians should be trained to dewax. Technicians responded mainly in the affirmative, with 77% of those asked answering 'Yes'. Consultants were evenly split on the issue, 50% of those replying thought this a good idea, and 50% thought the opposite. however, a large proportion of respondents, both technicians and consultants, deliberated over the question, particularly those responding in the affirmative, feeling the solution was not clear cut:

Table 30.5
Should technicians be
trained to dewax?

| | PERCENTAGE | |
	Technicians	Consultants
Yes	62	38
No	19	38
Missing information	19	25

*'I think we should look more broadly and if the technician knows about the
ear and are taught and trained about it and wax is a bar to them doing
what they're supposed to be doing and it's a procedure which somebody at
a sub-doctor level is capable of doing, the answer is yes' (consultant).*

30.6.2 A couple of technicians felt that they are in fact better qualified than
nurses who are frequently allowed to dewax:

*'Yes, in a way because we do similar things, probably just as well
qualified if not better than some of the nurses who do it, so yes I think we
should do it' (technician).*

*'They get their practice nurses to do it and as far as I know the practice
nurses have not had any training at all, no formal training by ENT staff on
dewaxing' (technician).*

30.6.3 Not everyone agreed on the methods of dewaxing that technicians
should be allowed to use. A number suggested only peripheral wax should be
removed, some felt syringing would be appropriate whilst others were
against technicians using syringing as a method of removing wax:

*'If that person wants training to dewax through syringing, not microscopic
work then yes I think it would be appropriate' (consultant).*

*'I think it would be nice if we were shown how to get a little tool and
scoop a bit of wax out of the bottom of the eardrum because quite often
you're looking down and you think if only that little lump wasn't
there....but as for syringing I wouldn't touch it with a bargepole, I mean
you can't see the eardrum, you don't know what state it's in' (technician).*

30.6.4 There were a variety of conditions stipulated and a number of problems foreseen, with very few technicians or consultants giving a simple
'yes'. The question of responsibility was widely recognised:

*'Well, its who's going to take the responsibility for what's under that wax
really is the problem' (technician).*

'It's a matter of considerable litigation' (consultant).

30.6.5 Others felt that adding dewax to the list of technicians duties would
only add to their workload unnecessarily:

'It wouldn't be a bad thing but we don't have enough time to do what we need to do anyway' (technician).

30.6.6 It was also pointed out that wax may hide other problems in the ear drum that would then be discovered by the technician, and that its removal could cause further problems:

'No, I think you need medical training to do it. Just one simple reason for that is that some people when they're dewaxed get tinnitus afterwards, that sort of thing and they associate that – 'well it was the doctor who did it' (technician).

31   Medical Responsibility

31.1 Who takes medical responsibility?
(table 31.1)

31.1.1 A variety of answers were given to this question. In the main, technicians believed that the consultant whom the patient was under would be responsible. Many consultants, however, felt that some, if not all, of the responsibility lay with the referring GP. The disagreements were largely because Centres had never properly addressed the question. Only one of the 21 Centres had taken legal advice on the issue.

Table 31.1

Who takes medical responsibility for directly referred patients?

	—— PERCENTAGE ——	
	Technicians	Consultants
Definitely the GP	10	19
Definitely the ENT consultant	52	25
Shared responsibility between ENT and the GP	5	19
Probably the ENT consultant	10	6
Probably the GP	5	6
Medical Directorate	5	0
Audiology Services Manager	5	0
Missing information	10	25

31.1.2 Of the technicians asked their opinion, 11 out of a total of 19 believed the consultant would be responsible. An additional 2 thought it would probably be the consultant but were not very sure. This is compared to 4 out of 14 consultants who felt the responsibility would be down to them alone:

> 'Theoretically .... the consultant does because although the GP makes the referral to the Hearing Aid Department nevertheless the Hearing Aid Department is under my jurisdiction and therefore my responsibility'

31.1.3 Another consultant suggested it would probably be down to the ENT consultant but was not very sure. Three consultants believed responsibility would be shared between the consultant and the GP (also the health authority in one case):

'The answer is we're both responsible, if you mean for the service, I am responsible, but for the patient I think the GP is responsible for each individual patient' (consultant).

31.1.4 Two technicians and three consultants definitely felt the GP was primarily responsible, whilst both another technician and consultant agreed it would probably be down to the GP:

'We can't be responsible for cases which we've never seen or been referred' (consultant).

31.1.5 One technician believed the audiology services manager was ultimately responsible, another the medical directorate, whilst a third believed it would be their health authority.

31.1.6 Only one Centre had contacted the health authority solicitors to discuss this question. The answer they were given was that:

'The health authority takes liability and responsibility for the actions of the staff employed by it ..... provided those actions fall within the remit of their job description. ....If you then do that (job) negligently then the authority is liable so far as the patient and public are concerned, but the authority may in the normal course of events have a disciplinary case against you' (technician).

31.1.7 The consultant in this Centre added to this by saying it was a shared responsibility because although the health authority would:

'Take ultimate responsibility for all employees, including me from the point of view if there was ever any kind of negligence leading to a pay-out......but if you like the management of the patient medically is down to me and the system which has been introduced in the department which I am responsible for in having done the assessment concerning the safety' (consultant).

Also:

'The GP also has a degree of responsibility and this is emphasised to him in the letter that they are going to be the only medical practitioner that the patient actually sees' (consultant).

31.1.8 In this Centre, the consultant had made sure that the examination of directly referred patients was made part of the technicians' job description so that in the case of any litigation arising, they would be covered by the health authority.

31.1.9 In none of the 21 Centres visited had litigation related to Direct Referral ever occurred. The medico-legal position of DR is discussed more fully in Part I, chapter 23.

32   Waiting Times

32.1 Waiting times
(tables 32.1, 32.2, 32.3)

32.1.1 Centres were asked what the typical waiting times from GP to examination, and from examination to fitting, were at present for both DR and TR patients. The two waits have been added together to give total waiting times from GP referral to hearing aid fitting. For various reasons there is missing data relating to the length of the waiting list for five of the Centres.

Table 32.1
Typical waiting times from
GP referral to fitting of aid

Centre	Traditional Referral	Direct Referral
1	14 weeks	9 weeks
2	16	8
3	34	13
4	12	5
5	#	16
6	28	#
7	63	17
8	38	#
9	26	13
10	#	#
11	32	14
12	24	4
13	#	28
14	28	22
15	26	40
16	18	14
17	30	9
18	44	68
19	21	16
20	19	5
21	12	8

\# = Not applicable or not known
Median waiting time for Traditional Referral is 26 weeks
Median waiting time for Direct referral is 13 weeks

32.1.2 For the majority of Centres the difference between DR and TR in the total length of wait is largely due to shorter waits under DR for the examination appointment. In contrast, there is little if any difference between times from examination to fitting for most of the Centres.

32.1.3 Data is complete for 16 out of the 21 Centres. For these Centres, total waiting times (i.e. from GP to fitting) for TR range from 12 weeks up to 63

Table 32.2
Typical waiting times from
GP referral to examination

Centre	Traditional Referral	Direct Referral
1	6 weeks	5 weeks
2	12	4
3	26	5
4	10	3
5	#	12
6	10	#
7	52	6
8	21	#
9	18	5
10	#	#
11	20	5
12	24	2
13	#	24
14	14	8
15	12	28
16	12	8
17	18	5
18	32	52
19	14	8
20	16	2
21	6	2

= Not applicable or not known.
Median waiting time for Traditional Referral is 15 weeks
Median waiting time for Direct Referral is 5 weeks

Table 32.3
Typical waiting times from
examination to fitting

Centre	Traditional Referral	Direct Referral
1	8 weeks	4 weeks
2	4	4
3	8	8
4	2	2
5	12	4
6	18	#
7	11	11
8	17	#
9	8	8
10	6	#
11	12	9
12	2	2
13	#	4
14	14	14
15	14	12
16	6	6
17	12	4
18	12	16
19	7	8
20	3	3
21	6	6

= Not applicable or not known
Median waiting time for Traditional Referral is 8 weeks
Median waiting time for Direct Referral is 6 weeks

weeks with 9 Centres having waits of 6 months or more. Under DR, the range is 4 weeks to 68 weeks, but the latter figure is exceptional, as only two Centres have a wait of 6 months or more. Overall, the median waiting time for DR is half of the wait for TR: 13 weeks compared to 26 weeks. Fourteen of these 16 Centres have a shorter length of wait to fitting under Direct Referral than under Traditional Referral. The difference ranges from 4 to 30 weeks.

32.1.4 At just 2 Centres the wait under DR is longer than under TR. At both these Centres the wait for DR patients is 14 weeks longer than for TR patients. At one, the situation is described as a temporary problem due largely to staff leaving:

'The reason for that is we lost our hearing therapist and I'm having to undertake the responsibility for the tinnitus patients and assessments so where I'd spend a fair amount of time organizing the DR clinics, unfortunately it's been put, not on hold, but its tended to increase the list. I see that as short term' (technician)

32.1.5 At the other Centre a combination of factors have led to the waiting list problem: staff posts have been frozen, the general workload including the number of directly referred patients have been increasing, and there has not been enough funding to provide the aids:

'In practice here I think we're looking at abnormal times, although our management will not have it, that's where we've been cut back because of going into Trust. I'm sure we've got to get our books in order and be in the black at the end of the financial year' (technician)

33 Problems, Benefits and Disadvantages of Direct Referral

33.1 Introduction

33.1.1 A number of issues relating to the operation of a DR system were listed under the three headings of 'Problems', 'Benefits', and 'Disadvantages'. These issues were believed to be important as they were topics repeatedly mentioned during preliminary interviews with staff at the 12 Centres where pilot Direct Referral schemes were set up (the subject of Part I of this report), and/or issues consequently raised during discussions on the progress of the schemes.

33.1.2 Under each of the three headings a list of items was drawn up and given to each person interviewed, who was asked to tick the most appropriate response to each item. The response categories were: (1) Major Problem (or Benefit or Disadvantage); (2) Minor Problem; (3) No Problem; (4) Don't Know. Missing information was rare using this method, although information was incomplete for the category 'problems at present' for the 3 Centres not running DR at the time of interview. All answers were calculated as a percentage, based upon the actual number of responses. In addition, interviewees were asked if there were any issues under these headings that had not been listed, if so these were discussed at greater length. The lists presented to technicians and consultants were considerably different, reflecting their different concerns and areas of knowledge.

33.1.3 The checklist concerned with any problems that had been encountered was answered with regard to both the past history of the DR scheme and the present situation. It was thought Centres that had been running DR for some length of time may have been able to resolve any initial problems they may have had.

33.2 Current problems – technicians
(table 33.1)

33.2.1 The main problems at the time of interviewing were, according to the technicians, the general workload (31% 'major', 25% 'minor'), and the number of patients needing a dewax (25% 'major', 44% 'minor'):

'The problem with the scheme in a sense is that its provided a much better arrangement to the patient but because of that the GP is far more aware that the facility now exists for them to bypass the consultant and they don't particularly want to use valuable ENT time so there's an increase in referrals'.

Table 33.1

Technician ratings of current problems with Direct Referral

Problem	Major	Minor	No problem	Don't know
A) The quality of Direct Referrals from GPs	6%	29%	65%	–
B) The number of Direct Referrals	19	25	56	–
C) Patient satisfaction with the scheme	–	6	94	–
D) The number of patients needing a dewax	25	44	31	–
E) The level of technician training or competence	–	12	88	–
F) Technicians opposing the scheme	–	–	100	–
G) ENT staff opposing the scheme	–	6	94	–
H) Funding the scheme	27	6	60	6
I) Day to day management of the scheme	–	6	94	–
J) Having staff to operate the scheme	18	24	59	–
k) The general workload	31	25	44	–
L) The number of patients being cross-referred	6	31	63	–

'The other worrying problem was to us the large number of patients, a significant proportion who needed dewax and given that we were running very short times between seeing the GPs and ourselves it was inconceivable to us the quantities of wax in some peoples ears'.

33.2.2 The number of DR patients, and having the staff to operate the scheme, are also felt to be major problems to 19% and 18% of technicians respectively and minor problems to an additional quarter of them:

'Recruitment – the biggest problems with the technicians is that there's a national shortage of them and everybody's tending to work understaffed at the moment'.

'I have 3 vacancies at the moment, the money's there, I just cannot recruit trained staff to the grade I want'.

33.2.3 The problem of unfilled vacancies appears widespread and national. There were vacancies for audiological staff at 9 out of 18 Centres where this information was available, and some, being unable to find suitable technicians, had resorted to filling vacancies with hearing and speech therapists instead.

33.2.4 Funding the scheme is seen as a major problem in over one quarter of all schemes (27%):

'Basically we were fitting more patients but they wouldn't give us any more money for hearing aids'.

One Centre feels that it is a minor problem, and 60% feel that it is no problem at all.

33.2.5 Although just one technician (in each case) felt that the quality of referrals from GPs and the number of patients being cross-referred to ENT were causing major problems, well over one quarter did have minor problems with these (29% and 31% respectively):

'Particular doctors who were persistent in their failure to refer adequately checked patients'.

'We're most particularly worried about the appearance of some of the pathologies and ears pouring with pus, large perforations, huge conductive hearing losses, this was something that did disturb us at the time and still does'.

33.2.6 A few staff (including consultants) were of the opinion that GPs were intentionally abusing the system by referring patients unsuitable for Direct Referral. This was in the knowledge that they would be referred on to a consultant within a short space of time, thereby bypassing the long waiting list for ENT.

33.2.7 The statement 'technicians opposing the scheme' met with a 100% response of 'no problem'. ENT staff opposing the scheme also had a very high percentage of technicians saying there was 'no problem' (94%). It can be argued however that Direct Referral is not likely to have been introduced in Centres where there was any great opposition to the scheme.

33.2.8 The day to day management of the scheme also had a very high percentage of technicians saying there is 'no problem' (94%). This was also true of patient satisfaction (94%) with a number of technicians commenting that satisfaction in fact appeared to have increased under DR:

'They're much more satisfied ... one technician usually starts or goes over their letter from their GP and it's so much more personal and individual, the same person checks their ears, asks them all these numerous questions, then takes the impression and gives them the little book, sometimes the same person even fits them.'

'If we contrast it with the ones we see through our normal procedure pattern they get a much better deal. I would say a hundred per cent better deal'.

33.2.9 One technician suggested an additional (unlisted) problem with Direct Referral was the extra length of time it took those patients who had to be cross-referred to ENT, to get their hearing aid.

33.3 Comparison of current problems with the past – technicians
(table 33.2)

33.3.1 As well as rating their current problems, technicians were also asked to rate whether any of these had been problems 'in the past'. Comparison of past and present problems shows that in many areas technicians were of the opinion that things had improved. Of particular note is the perceived improvement in the quality of referrals from GPs: 65% of technicians said that they are 'no problem' now compared with 32% who felt they were 'no problem' in the past. Just 6% (one technician) felt they were still a 'major problem' now compared with 21% in the past.

Table 33.2
Technician ratings of problems with Direct Referral in the past

Problem	Major	Minor	No problem	Don't know
A) The quality of Direct Referrals from GPs	21%	47%	32%	–
B) The number of Direct Referrals	22	28	44	6
C) Patient satisfaction with the scheme	–	11	90	–
D) The number of patients needing a dewax	39	44	17	–
E) The level of technician training or competence	–	28	72	–
F) Technicians opposing the scheme	–	5	90	5
G) ENT staff opposing the scheme	5	11	84	–
H) Funding the scheme	24	12	53	12
I) Day to day management of the scheme	–	39	61	–
J) Having staff to operate the scheme	32	32	37	–
k) The general workload	44	17	39	–
L) The number of patients being cross-referred	6	39	56	–

33.3.2 The major changes have been significant decreases in the numbers of technicians feeling that the following are a major problem:
a.   The quality of Direct Referrals (21% reduced to 6%)
b.   The number of patients needing a dewax (39% to 25%)
c.   Having the staff to operate the scheme (32% to 18%)
d.   The general workload (44% to 31%)

33.3.3 The numbers of technicians stating that the volume of DR patients and funding the scheme were a major problem has stayed constant. Finally, there does not appear to be any problems that have, on the whole, got worse over time.

33.4 Current problems – consultants
(table 33.3)

33.4.1 There are two problems causing major concern to consultants. Firstly, a lack of technicians (30% 'major', 30% 'minor'):

'If we've got a problem it would be the availability of trained technicians because training schemes are few'.

Table 33.3

Consultant ratings of
present problems with
Direct Referral

Problem	Major	Minor	No problem	Don't know
A) The number of DR patients being sent to ENT for dewax	15%	46%	39%	–
B) The level of technician training or competence	–	–	100	–
C) ENT staff opposing the scheme	–	7	93	–
D) The number of DR patients being cross-referred to ENT	–	8	92	–
E) Patients being re-referred by their GP for conditions not picked up by the technician	–	–	100	–
F) Demands placed on service by DR system interfering with technician support for ENT clinics	–	54	46	–
G) Not enough technicians	30	30	39	–

'We're in yet another financial noose at the moment which has twice reduced the number of technicians to the point of which it's going to affect service'.

33.4.2 Secondly, the number of DR patients being sent to ENT for a dewax (15% 'major' and 46% 'minor'):

'The fact is, many of our GPs simply are not even competent to look down an ear and recognise wax let alone anything more complex'

33.4.3 Whilst no consultants felt the demands placed upon the service by Direct Referral interfered with technician support for ENT clinics in a major way, over half did however rate this a minor problem:

'But there is a conflict of interest between Direct Referral and clinic support because the Direct Referral is the prime responsibility of the technicians and therefore is their priority because they are responsible for it........so when you have got a situation where everybody's sick then each department will think that theirs is a priority and they should have what few staff there are'.

33.4.4 No consultants felt there was a problem with the level of technician training or competence, or with regard to patients being re-referred by their GP for conditions not picked up by the technician.

**33.5 Comparison of
current problems with the
past – consultants**
(table 33.4)

33.5.1 On most issues, consultants indicated very little change over time in the number of problems reported. However, with regard to the important matter of the numbers of cross-referrals to ENT, some improvement over time was in evidence: whilst 20% of consultants felt this had been a minor problem in the past only 8% felt it to be a problem currently.

Table 33.4
Consultant ratings of
problems with Direct
Referral in the past

Problem	Major	Minor	No problem	Don't know
A) The number of DR patients being sent to ENT for dewax	17%	50%	33%	–
B) The level of technician training or competence	8	–	92	–
C) ENT staff opposing the scheme	–	8	92	–
D) The number of DR patients being cross-referred to ENT	–	20	80	–
E) Patients being re-referred by their GP for conditions not picked up by the technician	–	–	100	–
F) Demands placed on service by DR system interfering with technician support for ENT clinics	–	58	42	–
G) Not enough technicians	25	50	25	–

33.5.2 Whilst one consultant felt there was a major problem in the level of technician training in the past, this has been overcome through time. The consultant concerned was specifically referring to the lack of training in dewaxing:

'There has been no problem with competence and there's not a problem with competence now, there has been a problem with training which had to be addressed in the past, because that's this wax problem because we had to train them how to remove wax but that is not a problem now'.

33.6 Benefits – technicians
(table 33.5)

33.6.1 From the list of benefits shown to the head technicians there were four that were thought to be particularly important. These were:

a. A faster service to patients (75% 'major benefit').
b. The technicians job is more varied and interesting (75% 'major benefit').
c. Integration of the whole process of provision (74% 'major benefit').
d. A better quality service to patients (72% 'major benefit').

Table 33.5
Technician ratings of
benefits of Direct Referral

Benefit	Major	Minor	No benefit	Don't know
A) A faster service to patients	75%	10%	10%	5%
B) A better quality service to patients	72	17	11	–
C) Technicians job is more varied and interesting	75	20	5	–
D) Technicians feel more valued and respected	65	20	10	5
E) It is easier to develop community outreach services	53	21	26	–
F) More direct contact between Hearing Aid Centre and GPs	42	47	11	–
G) Provides a more personal service to patients as individuals	63	16	16	5
H) Integrates the whole process of provision	74	16	11	–

33.6.2 With regard to integrating the provision process, this was often seen as leading to an improvement in service efficiency:

'You can actually book your patients in better. The way we do it on the ENT clinics we do the impression at the same time as the audio, so if you've got a huge ENT clinic with people waiting and consultants jumping up and down because only one technician is doing hearing tests and you've got four people waiting outside for an impression it can cause problems.... when you do your own scheme you run very much to time so that patients are rarely kept waiting more than ten minutes so its much smoother running'.

33.6.3 The major reasons why DR was seen as improving the quality of service were to do with it providing a more 'personal' care and less hurried service:

'We get control of the patient right the way through in that they're seeing the same faces and we're possibly able to afford a little more time'.

'It is less traumatic coming directly to the department. We try and get them to see the same members of staff and identify with them, the ENT can be quite impersonal.... so I think we present a more caring front than entrance through an ENT department'.

' I think it's a better service because I think time is so important to the patients in if you do half an hour looking at their ears or whatever they're going to be happier than if they'd been in and out in a couple of seconds or minutes or so'.

33.6.4 Over half of the technicians interviewed believed Direct Referral had been a major benefit to them in developing community outreach services (53% 'major benefit') and that this in turn leads to a better quality of service to patients:

'The other advantage is you go and see patients in the environment in which they live so you can recommend any environmental aids they may need'

'I don't actually think they get a better quality in terms of technician potential if you like but they may well be better off in terms of surroundings and so on via the fact that they don't have to go so far geographically'

33.6.5 42% of technicians considered DR to be a major benefit in promoting more direct contact between the Hearing Aid Centre and GPs. Another 47% felt it was a minor benefit.

33.6.6 One additional benefit suggested by a couple of technicians was that a number of patients are reluctant to be examined by a consultant. Examination by an audiological technician as opposed to a consultant can be 'less stressful and traumatic for the elderly patients':

> *'The vast majority of people don't really want to go through an ENT major examination, all they do want is some kind of hearing aid'.*

> *'Many of them come round actually smarting from their experience with the ENT consultant'*

33.6.7 However one other technician did oppose this point of view:

> *'If a patient thinks they're coming to see a consultant generally speaking, initially there is a bit of disappointment'.*

33.6.8 Another suggested benefit of Direct Referral not covered by the checklist was:

> *'It gives more weight to the Audiology Department, they put them higher up in the hospital's list of priorities. If you're competing as part of ENT and looking for resources that are available within ENT they will tend to go more to the type of patients that the ENT surgeons themselves deal with.... in some ways they view hearing aid provision almost as a failure – 'here's one we can't do anything about'.*

33.7 Benefits – consultants
(table 33.6)

33.7.1 The single most important benefit of Direct Referral from the consultants' point of view has been the faster service to hearing aid patients. Out of 14 consultants from whom information was available, 13 rated this a 'major benefit', while the last did not think it had any benefit in this respect. However, information was missing from the one Centre which had permanently halted DR due to a long waiting list, and from 3 Centres that had suspended DR at some time; therefore the overall benefit may not be as great as this result suggests. Generally, DR does provide a faster service provided sufficient technical staff are available, but waiting lists can increase quickly in a situation of staff shortage.

Table 33.6
Consultant ratings of benefits of Direct Referral

Benefit	Major	Minor	No benefit	Don't know
A) A faster service to hearing aid patients	93%	–	7%	–
B) An improved service to other ENT patients	43	57	–	–
C) ENT time has been freed for more serious cases	62	23	15	–
D) ENT doctors have been relieved of seeing hearing aid patients they can do nothing for	50	36	14	–
E) Technicians have developed a more professional attitude to their work	58	8	8	25

33.7.2 Removal of patients from the ENT queue as a result of DR has a number of additional benefits for ENT. All of the consultants felt that the service to other ENT patients had improved as a result, to some degree, and most acknowledged that ENT time had been freed for more serious cases (62% 'major benefit', 23% 'minor benefit').

33.7.3 58% of consultants thought that a major benefit of DR had been that technicians had developed a more professional attitude to their work:

> *'But I would say it has made a difference in the attitudes of the technicians to patients and GPs. They've had more direct contact with the GPs and therefore it's improved their professional status and attitude, yes'.*

However, one quarter said they did not know whether this had occurred or not, and a few did not like the question – saying that their technicians had a professional attitude even before DR.

33.7.4 No benefits other than those listed were suggested by consultants.

33.8 Disadvantages – technicians
(table 33.7)

33.8.1 The extra paperwork generated for the Hearing Aid Centre by Direct Referral was the only disadvantage that technicians as a group regarded as of any real concern. Nearly three quarters felt it was a disadvantage with 22% stating it was a 'major disadvantage'.

33.8.2 Only two other items received any 'major disadvantage' ratings: a) service to non DR patients has become poorer; and b) other aspects of audiology work have suffered. These were rated 'major' by just one technician (the same one), and the problems here had arisen due to time pressures.

33.8.3 Two items were concerned with involvement of consultants in the provision process: a) Direct Referral patients not receiving the benefit of an ENT consultant's expertise, and b) a loss of input from consultants on the

Table 33.7
Technician ratings of disadvantages of Direct Referral

Disadvantage	Major	Minor	No dis've	Don't know
A) The extra paperwork generated for the Hearing Aid Centre	22%	50%	22%	6%
B) DR patients do not receive the benefit of an ENT consultant's expertise	–	17	72	11
C) Loss of input from consultants on type of aid to be fitted	–	–	94	6
D) Service to non-DR patients has become poorer	6	11	72	11
E) Other aspects of Audiology Department work have suffered due to concentration on DR	6	11	72	11

type of aid to be fitted. None of the technicians considered either of these to be a disadvantage:

'I don't think you'll find many ENT consultants who've got very much expertise in prescribing hearing aids'.

'When it was just a B11 they would write it down but their attitude is why have a dog and bark yourself'.

'Because the consultants don't really know, you've just got the consultants sort of hierarchy as being God and saying what I say goes instead of passing it back on to professional people and letting them make the judgement'.

33.8.4 Another disadvantage noted by a couple of technicians was that not only do GPs off-load patients with ear problems to the Hearing Aid Department through the DR scheme, but some consultants do as well:

'I think the consultants were so anxious to offload their patients that if it said 'hearing aid' on the letter it was thrown to the DR clinic regardless'.

33.8.5 Another disadvantage with DR occurs when patients cannot be seen immediately in ENT if they have to be cross-referred. An extra journey for the patient in addition to an increase in waiting time may be the result.

33.8.6 This may also occur with patients that need wax removal where there are no facilities for them to be dewaxed at the time of appointment:

'They sometimes have to be sent away and then that's a waste of our time, the patients time, ambulance time'.

33.8.7 One technician spoke of a greater number of patients failing to keep appointments when they are directly referred:

'I think it's in the minds of some patients it might be slightly less important because it's not a doctor'.

**33.9 Disadvantages –
consultants**
(table 33.8)

33.9.1 From the ENT point of view the greatest disadvantage associated with DR was that doctors have become distanced from the hearing aid side of ENT work. 15% of consultants felt this a major disadvantage whilst 46% felt it a minor disadvantage:

'I think that this is, if it becomes more available that we are going to have fewer doctors interested in hearing aid work. As it is there are few enough who have any interest. But again, I think it's important that as ENT specialists we should know how to manage it, and I think it's an area that is sadly neglected in training'.

Table 33.8

Consultant ratings of disadvantages of Direct Referral

Disadvantage	Major	Minor	No dis'vge	Don't know
A) DR patients do not receive the benefit of an ENT consultant's expertise	–	23%	77%	–
B) Loss of input from consultants on the type of aid to be fitted	–	23	77	–
C) ENT doctors have become distanced from hearing aid side of ENT work	15	46	39	–
D) Service to non-DR hearing aid patients has become poorer	–	–	100	–
E) Other aspects of Audiology Department work have suffered due to concentration on DR	–	29	64	7

33.9.2 Another consultant argued that because 'their involvement was so minimal' prior to DR, it has made little difference.

33.9.3 No consultant had experienced the service to non-DR hearing aid patients becoming poorer. One in fact suggested that DR had resulted in a better service to these patients:

'I think the effect of Direct Referral has been to make all the technicians more interested in hearing aid fittings and made them feel more responsible, so I think in fact the actual standards of work has particularly gone up all round'.

33.9.4 Whilst the majority of consultants had not experienced the remaining two disadvantages on the list, approximately one quarter of them felt each had been a minor disadvantage. In reply to the item 'Direct Referral patients do not receive the benefit of an ENT consultant's expertise':

'I'd say minimum – some of the patients may wish to ask about their actual disability in terms of medical things, what has gone wrong and so forth'

And with regard to the item 'Other aspects of Audiology Department work have suffered due to concentration on DR':

'Until recently the answer would have been no but there is no doubt that the overall work of the department is building up, it's enormous'.

33.9.5 No disadvantages other than those on the checklist were mentioned.

34 The Benefits of DR Weighed Against the Disadvantages

34.1 Views of technicians

34.1.1 The great majority of technicians interviewed were enthusiastic about Direct Referral. Out of 17 that were asked outright, 16 said that the benefits of DR outweighed any disadvantages that may have occurred:

'Benefits – enormous!'

'I don't think we'd do it any other way'

'I find here that there are no problems whatsoever – in fact everybody, I think, benefits from it - technicians, patients, family, everybody'.

34.1.2 The one technician who did not express enthusiasm felt that in theory Direct Referral is a good idea but at present his Centre was running DR in 'abnormal times':

'Well, I've had posts frozen, I've been using locums which I've never used on Direct Referrals, and I had maternity leaves and the general things to make Direct Referral a bit difficult, or any scheme'.

34.1.3 Four technicians were not asked the question directly nevertheless they all expressed a positive attitude towards DR. Of the technicians interviewed in the two Centres where Direct Referral had stopped permanently one expressed a wish to reintroduce DR whilst the other still believed it had the potential to be a good system:

'I still, given the time, space and the staff, I say it's a good idea if it works well'.

34.2 Views of consultants

34.2.1 Most of the consultants interviewed were enthusiastic about Direct Referral. Out of 13 asked directly 9 replied positively:

'Oh yes, without a doubt'.

'Yes – definitely'.

34.2.2 A further 3 stipulated that subject to certain conditions, such as the availability and ability of technicians and the full support of ENT backup staff, the benefits can outweigh the disadvantages:

> *'Only if you have got properly trained technicians, an accessible ENT service and the kind of structure which allows individual appointments in the way that you do it. I think Direct Referral is diabolical if it is a cop-out with a student or basic grade doing it without direct access to consultants'.*

34.2.3 Just one of the consultants interviewed had a generally negative view of DR. This particular consultant had experience of working within 2 Centres that used DR. Whilst one of the schemes was felt to be running satisfactorily, the other was not – this was due primarily to the quality of referrals and the ability of the staff involved.

34.2.4 It is also important to note that information was missing from 3 of the interviews, in addition to the Centres where the consultants were not interviewed. As this includes both the Centres which had stopped DR and a further 2 where it had been suspended at some stage it is likely that the information from the consultants available for interview is not fully representative.

35 Advice for those thinking of Setting up DR Schemes

35.1 Advice offered by technicians and consultants

35.1.1 In response to the question 'What advice would you give to somebody who was thinking of starting a DR system?', a wide variety of recommendations were made. The suggestions made can conveniently be divided into four main categories: GP involvement, ENT, technical staff, and organisation of the scheme.

35.2 Advice – GP involvement

35.2.1 Technicians in particular spoke of the need for greater GP awareness of what Direct Referral actually involves. Many suggested that GPs need some form of training to ensure that they refer appropriate patients, in particular patients without wax:

> *'I would certainly advise that they teach their GPs well and give them concrete instruction if you like, about what criteria would be acceptable, age limits, the fact that it's no use sending somebody if they've got a discharge or an ear blocked up with wax' (technician).*

35.2.2 Giving the GPs a comprehensive set of criteria was also judged to be important. One of the technicians felt it would be a good idea to include some of the GPs in the compiling of the criteria for the referral form:

> *'It was chosen because it had been recommended, incorporated guidelines laid down by the Hearing Aid Council and the TTSA, but in actual fact when it came to putting it into practice we found that there are a proportion of the questions which are consistently useless or the GPs are consistently inaccurate or poor in their ability to answer the questions appropriately' (technician).*

35.2.3 It was stressed that a good relationship with GPs was particularly beneficial as was direct contact when problems arise at either end.

35.2.4 There was some difference of opinion over what to do with patients inappropriately referred by GPs: whether to cross directly to ENT or to send such patients straight back to their GP:

'Communicate back to the GPs and if you do end up cross referring the patient write back to the GP and tell him you've cross referred the patient and with a bit of luck he will work out that it's a waste of time sending the referrals in and he'll send them to the right place in the first place' (technician).

'If they send somebody that had a simple problem they should just be sent back to them, the patient would have to go back to the beginning of the queue again, then they (GPs) might behave' (consultant).

35.2.5 Whichever way this problem is dealt with, it is important to recognise that inappropriate referrals will occur and to prepare for this eventuality:

'If you're not expecting to have ENT referrals amongst your hearing aid lot, you immediately run into difficulties about what to do with them at the time but if you've got yourself organised that you know what to do with them if you do find them it's OK, it doesn't seem to be a problem as far as we're concerned here' (technician).

35.3 Advice – ENT

35.3.1 The second major area covered by the advice concerned the ENT department. Both technicians and consultants suggested the need of adequate ENT support for DR. The technicians must feel confident that they can refer on to ENT any patient they are unsure or unhappy about:

'You've got to have an absolute guarantee out of the ENT consultant that they will take patients as an emergency, they are going to take seriously anyone you refer to the clinic and must treat that as emergency and priority' (technician).

'Obviously you've got to have co-operation of ENT people, you've got to have some sort of backing, if you do find problems or run into difficulties, there's no point in setting it up and then finding that you're inundated with ENT problems and nobody is prepared to take them off your hands, so you have to make sure that other people who are involved or could be involved are going to be supportive really'. (technician)

'If there's any doubts about it in the ENT dept between colleagues, it could give rise to problems, particularly if there's litigations'. (consultant)

35.3.2 This last point was further reiterated by another consultant who did suggest it would be wise to establish the legal position of medical responsibility before starting Direct Referral.

35.4 Advice – technical staff

35.4.1 The third major area of advice concerned the technicians themselves. Not only was ENT approval needed for a successful DR scheme but technician support was also important:

'If they're unhappy and feel the responsibility is too great they shouldn't be forced to use it' (consultant).

'Make sure that staff are au fait with the idea and are quite happy working with it' (consultant).

35.4.2 In addition, the technicians need to be competent and experienced:

'You've got to know what your staff are capable of' (technician).

'Make sure that you're happy to take your responsibility checking ears or reading patient's history but in the main just know your subject and then you won't go too far wrong' (technician).

35.4.3 There also needs to be enough staff to cover the clinics, particularly in the eventuality that Direct Referral may lead to increased referrals.

35.5 Advice – organization

35.5.1 The final major area of advice was to do with organization of the scheme:

'Organize it first, think it through, organize the time, clerical staff, how they're going to run the clinics, how they're going to structure the clinics, everything about it before they just go and do it' (technician).

35.5.2 A number of technicians felt that an awareness of time management was important:

'It's a temptation to try to overbook (so that time is not wasted when a patient does not attend) and then of course everyone arrives so it's a bit like a cattle market and the timing is crucial' (technician).

'You've got to build in equivalent times for seeing these patients afterwards as well, you can't say they're a one off, we'll see them as a GP referral, you have got to allow time to see them afterwards for a fitting, for a follow up and for repairs' (technician).

'However much time you allow is never quite enough, there are always more problems than you think of' (technician).

35.5.3 Making sure that you have enough man-hours (particularly clerical time) for administration tasks was also felt to be very important.

35.5.4 A number of technicians suggested there was a need to build the system up slowly so that problems can be tackled as and when they occur:

'Try it on a softly-softly approach and not on the blatant – here we are, we can take it from any GP - just to let the odd GP know.'

'Feel your way, say to yourself we're going to have 6 to 9 months of getting this organized, having one or two referrals a week, half a dozen a month and watch it and see what happens because if you do come across problems in other areas that you just haven't anticipated, if you're doing it that way, you've got the time, the ability, the knowledge to sort that problem out.'

35.5.5 It was also suggested that a certain level of resources is needed before DR can be implemented. This includes the hearing aids themselves, equipment for testing and the rooms:

'I know of departments who still work from virtually a cupboard and to try to develop a DR system from such a thing is asking too much of the technicians' (consultant).

35.5.6 A couple of technicians suggested it would be beneficial for anyone thinking of starting Direct Referral to look round a hospital where DR was in operation:

'So to come in and actually for them to see how your system works and then try to relate that to what they plan to do, what they would do in a different way'

35.6 Advice – other

35.6.1 Other advice included keeping Direct Referral to older age groups:

'Any young adult losing hearing for no reason should be seen as a matter of urgency in my view, no way do I want that kind of patient, absolutely no way' (technician).

35.7 Also, keeping the waiting list down:

'Paramount importance is to keep the list down, even if it means doing a double clinic one week' (technician).

'The important thing is to keep on, even if it hurts a bit at the time because there's no doubt about it why the main purpose of Direct Referral is to keep the time down and it defeats the object if you're going to allow yourself to build up a waiting list' (technician).

35.7.1 Finally, a couple of consultants kept the advice short and to the point: 'proceed'.

Questionnaire used in postal survey of all Hearing Aid Centres in England

Hester Adrian Research Centre

from:

David Reeves

Tel 061 275 3536
Fax 061 275 3333

The University
Manchester M13 9PL
United Kingdom

Director Professor Chris Kiernan BA PhD

D. J. Reeves
18th February 1991

Dear Sir or Madam,

DEPARTMENT OF HEALTH HEARING AID SERVICES PROJECT

Please find enclosed a short questionnaire about any schemes of ACCELERATED REFERRAL or DIRECT REFERRAL for hearing aid provision which you may operate at your Centre. This is part of a national survey being conducted by ourselves (HARC), in the context of an evaluation of direct referral practices in this country commissioned by the Department of Health. For more information, please see the Department of Health Executive Letter No EL(90)P/9 dated 15th January 1990 from Mr K S Jacobson addressed to District General Managers and copied to Regional and District Chairmen and Regional General Managers.

The questionnaire is very brief and will only take a few minutes to complete. A stamped addressed envelope is enclosed for your reply. Please note that it is *equally* important that you respond if you do not operate these procedures, as one of our concerns is to identify the extent of these procedures relative to total provision. If you do not operate either procedure, the questionnaire will literally take only seconds to complete.

If you feel that you have already supplied some of this information in the context of a previous survey connected with this project (February 1990), please accept our apologies, but we would nonetheless be grateful if you would complete this more specific questionnaire.

Please return the completed questionnaire by *14th March 1991*.

Yours faithfully,

D. J. Reeves

Hearing Aid Services Project
Survey of Direct and Accelerated Referral Practices

Centre:

Your name _____

Position _____

On average, approximately how many *new patients*
does your Centre (including peripheral clinics) fit
with hearing aids each month   _____

For each of the following forms of referral for a hearing aid, please indicate the situation in your centre:

1. ACCELERATED REFERRAL
   The patient's GP writes to a consultant in the ENT department. The
   consultant (or other appropriate doctor) decides on the basis of the letter
   whether the patient requires an ENT examination or not. Where he/she
   feels that examination is *not* necessary, he/she cross-refers the patient
   straight to the hearing aid department for assessment and fitting.

   Do you use this procedure at all?

   ☐ No   ☐ Yes   ☐ Have in the Past   ☐ Intend to in the Future

2. DIRECT REFERRAL
   The patient's GP writes directly to the hearing aid department, asking
   that the patient be assessed/fitted with a hearing aid. The patient is not
   seen by an ENT consultant or other doctor unless the audiology
   technicians feel that it is necessary.

   Do you use this procedure at all?

   ☐ No   ☐ Yes   ☐ Have in the Past   ☐ Intend to in the Future

   └──────── PLEASE ANSWER THE QUESTIONS OVERLEAF

217

The following questions are only for those who operate or have operated Direct Referral (DR)

If you currently operate DR, on average roughly how many new patients are directly referred to you each month _____

Roughly how many of these are straight-forward hearing aid fittings with no complications (e.g. do not need to be cross-referred to ENT or sent back to their GP) _____

Date that DR began _____

Date that DR ended (if applicable) _____

Reasons for ending DR (if applicable) _____
_____
_____
_____

Sites at which DR is/was in operation _____
_____
_____
_____

Any additional comments _____
_____
_____
_____

Name and address of who we may contact (if not yourself) for further information on the DR system
Name_____
Address_____
_____ Tel_____

If you have produced any documents pertaining to audit or assessment of your DR system, we would be very grateful to receive copies of these.

Return to: Hearing Aid Services Project, HARC, The University,
            Oxford Rd., Manchester M13 9PL

If you have any queries about this questionnaire, please contact
            David Reeves, HARC, tel 061–275–3536

Appendix II.II

Interview schedules used with technicians and consultants at selected centres

Note 1:   All interviews were recorded and transcribed

Note 2:   The interview schedules provided here are the versions used with Centres that had never stopped or suspended their DR scheme. The versions used with the latter were basically the same, but with minor modifications.

AUDIOLOGIST INTERVIEWS – DIRECT REFERRAL SCHEMES
SURVEY
Continuous schemes

Hospital _____

Interviewer _____

Date _____

Audiologist _____

Read the following statement to the interviewee:

The purpose of this interview is to find out what your experience has been of operating a Direct Referral system. Thus in the course of the interview we will be particularly interested in how your system is organised, the benefits you feel it provides, and any problems you have experienced in running the system. The information you give will be used to benefit other centres which may be thinking of introducing Direct Referral.

Anything you say will be treated completely confidentially and will not be attributed to either you personally or to your centre in any report or publication.

Part 1 (Background information)

Job Title _____

Grade – MTO _____ Other _____

Years in current post _____

Number of staff in dept:

	In post	Vacant
Audiological Scientist	_____	_____
Technician (senior)	_____	_____
Technician (junior)	_____	_____
Hearing Therapist	_____	_____
Speech Therapist	_____	_____

Current Waiting Times (average)

Traditional Referral (i.e. via ENT clinic examination)

GP	– ENT examination	_____
ENT	– Impression	_____
Imp	– Fitting	_____

Direct Referral

GP	– DR examination	_____
DR exam	– Impression	_____
Imp	– Fitting	_____

Do you operate a hearing aid clinic* ?   1. Yes   2. No

IF YES – ASK FOR WAITING TIMES

Hearing Aid clinic waiting times
    GP   – Examination   _____
    Exam   – Impression   _____
    Imp   – Fitting   _____

(* A hearing aid clinic is where GPs send referral letters to either an ENT consultant or the Hearing Aid Department. Those patients thought to only need a hearing aid attend a special clinic session where they are checked by an ENT doctor (typically a junior) before the ear impressions are taken).

Part 2 (Organisation of the DR system)
1) How many technicians are involved in examining DR patients at present?

Does this include private dispensers?

1. Yes   2. No
   IF YES – how many?_____

What form of contract do you have with the private dispensers?

1. Employed on same basis as NHS technicians
2. Paid a standard rate for each patient seen / fitted
3. Paid a standard rate per hour spent with DR patient.
4. Other _____

2) What grades are the technicians examining DR patients?

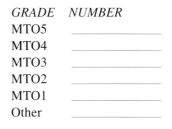

GRADE	NUMBER
MTO5	_____
MTO4	_____
MTO3	_____
MTO2	_____
MTO1	_____
Other	_____

3) Is there a minimum grade or number of years experience for a technician to reach before they examine Direct Referral patients

1. Yes   2. No
   IF YES – specify _____

4) At which of the following sites are DR patients seen?

Main hospital_____ 1. Yes 2. No
Peripheral hospital/clinics_____ 1. Yes 2. No
Domiciliary visits_____ 1. Yes 2. No
Other community settings
(eg old peoples homes)_____ 1. Yes 2. No

5) Is there a minimum age for Direct Referral patients?

1. Yes 2. No
    IF YES – specify_____(years)

6) Do the GPs send referral letters directly to the audiology dept?

1. Yes 2. No

7) Do the consultants cross-refer patients on the basis of the GP letter ? (ie the patient is not seen by an ENT doctor)

1. Yes 2. No

8) Were you here when the Direct Referral scheme started up?

1. Yes 2. No
    IF YES – were you involved in implementing the scheme?
    IF YES – what did that entail?

9) What were the reasons behind the introduction of Direct Referral?

10) How were GPs made aware of the scheme?

   1. Mailshot to all/most GPs in area
   2. Individual GPs contacted personally
   3. Don't Know
   4. Other _____

11) Was there any training or presentation etc offered to the GPs?

   1. Yes 2. No 3. Don't Know
    IF YES – what did this consist of?
    IF YES – what was the attendance like out of the GPs invited?
    IF YES – was it successful?

12) Were GPs provided with a set of criteria to follow in order to select suitable patients for Direct Referral?

   1. Yes 2. No 3. Don't Know

13) Do the technicians use a standard set of criteria when examining Direct Referral patients?

1. Yes   2. No
IF YES – may we have a copy of the criteria

14) Is any special or additional training given to technicians who are going to be involved in examining DR patients?

1. Yes   2. No
IF YES – what form does this take?

15) What happens if the technician discovers something abnormal about a DR patients ear or pattern of loss.

1. Patient is cross-referred to ENT
2. Patient is referred back to GP
3. Other _____

16) Do any of the technicians ever do a dewax?

1. Yes – syringe only
2. Yes – more than syringe
3. No
   IF YES – who takes medical responsibility for the dewaxing?
   IF NO – do you think that technicians should be trained to dewax?
   1. Yes – but syringe only
   2. Yes – more than syringe
   3. No

17) Who takes medical responsibility for directly referred patients?

1. Definitely the GP
2. Probably the GP
3. Definitely the ENT consultant
4. Probably the ENT consultant
5. Don't Know
6. Other _____

18) Have you had any Direct Referral cases where medical responsibility has been important? (eg if a condition has been missed by the technician resulting in a compensation claim by the patient)

Part 3 (Opinions on the operation of the system)

19) I now want to ask some questions about problems you may have experienced with your Direct Referral scheme. This is a list of potential problems you may have experienced. (GIVE LIST 1). For each one, indicate how much of a problem it has been for your service. Please rate a problem as MAJOR if it has been a major problem *at any time*.

CONTINUE AFTER LIST 1 HAS BEEN COMPLETED.

20) Have you at any time experienced any major problems not on that list

    1. Yes   2. No
    IF YES – what problems

(Interviewer: at your discretion, discuss any problems rated as major)

21) I now want to ask you some questions about possible benefits of your Direct Referral system compared to standard referral practice. This is a list of possible benefits. (GIVE LIST 2). For each one, indicate how much of a benefit you think it has been for your service.

CONTINUE AFTER LIST 2 HAS BEEN COMPLETED

22) Have you experienced any major benefits that are not on that list?

    1. Yes   2. No
    IF YES – what benefits

(Interviewer: at your discretion discuss any benefits rated as major)

23) The next set of questions are concerned with disadvantages your DR system may have compared to traditional referral practice. This is a list of possible disadvantages. (GIVE LIST 3) indicate for each one how much of a disadvantage it has been in your service:

CONTINUE AFTER LIST 3 HAS BEEN COMPLETED

24) Are you aware of any disadvantages which are not on that list?

    1. Yes   2. No
    IF YES – what disadvantages

(Interviewer: at your discretion, discuss anything rated as major)

25) Overall, do you feel that the benefits of DR outweigh the disadvantages, or vice versa?

    1. Benefits outweigh   2. Disadvantages outweigh   3. Don't Know

26) Could the system be improved in any way?

    1. Yes   2. No
    IF YES – How?

27) Are you planning any changes in the Direct Referral system?

    1. Yes   2. No
    IF YES – What changes?

28) What advice would you give to somebody who was thinking of starting a Direct Referral system?

HAVE YOU HAD PROBLEMS WITH THE FOLLOWING IN CONNECTION WITH YOUR DIRECT REFERRAL SCHEME

Maj = This has been a major problem for us

Min = This has been a minor problem for us

No = This has not really been a problem for us

DK = I do not know if this has been a problem for us

	IN THE PAST				NOW			
a) The quality of Direct Referrals from GPs_____	Maj	Min	No	DK	Maj	Min	No	DK
b) The number of Direct Referrals_	Maj	Min	No	DK	Maj	Min	No	DK
c) Patient satisfaction with the DR scheme_____	Maj	Min	No	DK	Maj	Min	No	DK
d) Number of DR patients needing a dewax_____	Maj	Min	No	DK	Maj	Min	No	DK
e) Level of technician training or competence_____	Maj	Min	No	DK	Maj	Min	No	DK
f) Technicians opposing the DR scheme_____	Maj	Min	No	DK	Maj	Min	No	DK
g) ENT staff opposing the scheme_								
h) Funding the scheme_____	Maj	Min	No	DK	Maj	Min	No	DK
i) Day to day management of the scheme_____	Maj	Min	No	DK	Maj	Min	No	DK
j) Having Staff to operate the scheme_____	Maj	Min	No	DK	Maj	Min	No	DK
k) General workload_____	Maj	Min	No	DK	Maj	Min	No	DK
l) The number of DR patients being cross-referred to ENT_____	Maj	Min	No	DK	Maj	Min	No	DK

HAVE YOU EXPERIENCED ANY OF THE BELOW BENEFITS FROM OPERATING A DIRECT REFERRAL SCHEME

Maj = This has been a major benefit of our DR scheme

Min = This has been a minor benefit of our DR scheme

No = This has never really been a benefit of our DR scheme

DK = I do not know if this has been a benefit to us

a)   A faster service to patients _____   Maj   Min   No   DK

b)   A better quality service to patients _____   Maj   Min   No   DK

c)   Technicians job more interesting and varied _____   Maj   Min   No   DK

d)   Technicians feel more valued and respected _____   Maj   Min   No   DK

e)   Easier to develop community outreach services _____   Maj   Min   No   DK

f)   More direct contact between the hearing aid centre
     and GPs _____   Maj   Min   No   DK

g)   Provides a more personal service to patients as
     individuals _____   Maj   Min   No   DK

h)   Integrates the whole process of provision _____   Maj   Min   No   DK

HAVE YOU EXPERIENCED ANY OF THE BELOW DISADVANTAGES AS A RESULT OF OPERATING A DIRECT REFERRAL SCHEME

Maj = This has been a major disadvantage of our DR scheme

Min = This has been a minor disadvantage of our DR scheme

No = This has never really been a disadvantage of our DR scheme

DK = I do not know if this has been a disadvantage to us

a) The extra paperwork generated for the hearing aid
    centre_____   Maj Min No DK

b) DR Patients do not receive the benefit of the ENT
    consultants expertise_____   Maj Min No DK

c) Loss of input from consultants on type of aid to be
    fitted _____   Maj Min No DK

d) Service to non-DR patients has become poorer _____   Maj Min No DK

e) Other aspects of audiology departments work have
    suffered due to concentration on DR_____   Maj Min No DK

CONSULTANT INTERVIEWS – DIRECT REFERRAL SCHEMES
SURVEY
Continuous schemes

Hospital _____

Interviewer _____

Date_____

Consultant _____

Read the following statement to the interviewee:

The purpose of this interview is to find out what your experience has been of operating a Direct Referral system. Thus in the course of the interview we will be particularly interested in how your system is organised, the benefits you feel it provides, and any problems you have experienced in running the system. The information you give will be used to benefit other centres which may be thinking of introducing Direct Referral.

Anything you say will be treated completely confidentially and will not be attributed to either you personally or to your centre in any report or publication.

Part 1 (Background information)
Job Title _____

Years in current post_____

Number of ENT Consultants in the dept. _____

Number of Audiological Physicians in the dept. _____

Part two (Organisation of the scheme)
1) Were you here when the Direct Referral scheme started up?

    1. Yes 2. No
    IF YES – were you involved in implementing the scheme?
    IF YES – what did that entail?

2) What were the reasons behind the introduction of Direct Referral?

3) How were GPs made aware of the scheme?

    1. Mailshot to all/most GPs in area
    2. Individual GPs contacted personally
    3. Don't Know
    4. Other _____

4) Was there any training or presentation etc offered to the GPs?

    1. Yes 2. No 3. Don't Know
    IF YES – what did this consist of?
            – what was the attendance like out of the GPs invited?
            – was it successful?

5) Were GPs provided with a set of criteria to follow in order to select suitable patients for Direct Referral?

1. Yes   2. No   3. Don't Know

6) How confident do you feel that the technicians are referring on to the ENT dept all of the patients that need to be seen by an ENT doctor?

7) Have you undertaken any exercises to evaluate the performance of the technicians? (eg, examining a selection of DR patients they have fitted)

8) Who takes medical responsibility for directly referred patients?

1. Definitely the GP
2. Probably the GP
3. Definitely the ENT consultant
4. Probably the ENT consultant
5. Don't Know
6. Other _____

9) Have you had any Direct Referral cases where medical responsibility has been important? (eg if a condition has been missed by the technician resulting in a compensation claim by the patient)

Part 3 (Opinions on the operation of the system)

10) I now want to ask some questions about problems you may have experienced with your Direct Referral scheme. This is a list of potential problems you may have experienced. (GIVE LIST 1). For each one, indicate how much of a problem it has been for your service. Please rate a problem as MAJOR if it has been a major problem *at any time*.

CONTINUE AFTER LIST 1 HAS BEEN COMPLETED.

11) Have you at any time experienced any major problems not on that list

1. Yes   2. No
IF YES – what problems

(Interviewer: at your discretion, discuss any problems rated as major)

12) I now want to ask you some questions about possible benefits of your Direct Referral system compared to standard referral practice. This is a list of possible benefits. (GIVE LIST 2). For each one, indicate how much of a benefit you think it has been for your service.

CONTINUE AFTER LIST 2 HAS BEEN COMPLETED

13) Have you experienced any major benefits that are not on that list?

1. Yes   2. No
IF YES – what benefits

(Interviewer: at your discretion discuss any benefits rated as major)

14) The next set of questions are concerned with disadvantages your DR system may have compared to traditional referral practice. This is a list of possible disadvantages. (GIVE LIST 3) Indicate for each one how much of a disadvantage it has been in your service:

CONTINUE AFTER LIST 3 HAS BEEN COMPLETED

15) Are you aware of any disadvantages which are not on that list?

1. Yes   2. No
IF YES – what disadvantages

(Interviewer: at your discretion, discuss anything rated as major)

16) Overall, do you feel that the benefits of DR outweigh the disadvantages, or vice versa?

1. Benefits outweigh   2. Disadvantages outweigh   3. Don't Know

17) Could the system be improved in any way?

1. Yes   2. No
IF YES – How?

18) Do you think that technicians should be trained to dewax?

1. Yes – syringe only
2. Yes – more than syringe
3. No

19) What advice would you give to somebody who was thinking of starting a Direct Referral system?

HAVE YOU HAD PROBLEMS WITH THE FOLLOWING IN CONNECTION WITH YOUR DIRECT REFERRAL SCHEME

Maj = This has been a major problem for us

Min = This has been a minor problem for us

No = This has not really been a problem for us

DK = I do not know if this has been a problem for us

	IN THE PAST				NOW			
a) Number of DR patients being sent to ENT for dewax_____	Maj	Min	No	DK	Maj	Min	No	DK
b) Level of technician training or competence _____	Maj	Min	No	DK	Maj	Min	No	DK
c) ENT staff opposing the scheme _	Maj	Min	No	DK	Maj	Min	No	DK
d) The number of DR patients being cross-referred to ENT_____	Maj	Min	No	DK	Maj	Min	No	DK
e) Patients being re-referred by their GP for conditions not picked up by the technician _____	Maj	Min	No	DK	Maj	Min	No	DK
f) Demands placed on service by DR system interfering with technician support for ENT clinics_____	Maj	Min	No	DK	Maj	Min	No	DK
g) Not enough technicians_____	Maj	Min	No	DK	Maj	Min	No	DK

HAVE YOU EXPERIENCED ANY OF THE BELOW BENEFITS FROM OPERATING A DIRECT REFERRAL SCHEME

Maj = This has been a major benefit of our DR scheme

Min = This has been a minor benefit of our DR scheme

No = This has never really been a benefit of our DR scheme

DK = I do not know if this has been a benefit to us

a) A faster service to hearing aid patients _____ Maj Min No DK

b) An improved service to other ENT patients _____ Maj Min No DK

c) ENT time has been freed for more serious cases _____ Maj Min No DK

d) ENT doctors have been relieved of seeing hearing aid
    patients they can do nothing for_____ Maj Min No DK

e) Technicians have developed a more professional
    attitude to their work_____ Maj Min No DK

HAVE YOU EXPERIENCED ANY OF THE BELOW DISADVANTAGES AS A RESULT OF OPERATING A DIRECT REFERRAL SCHEME

Maj = This has been a major disadvantage of our DR scheme

Min = This has been a minor disadvantage of our DR scheme

No = This has never really been a disadvantage of our DR scheme

DK = I do not know if this has been a disadvantage to us

a) DR Patients do not receive the benefit of the ENT consultants expertise_____ Maj   Min   No   DK

b) Loss of input from consultants on type of aid to be fitted _____ Maj   Min   No   DK

c) ENT doctors have become distanced from hearing aid side of ENT work _____ Maj   Min   No   DK

d) Service to non-DR hearing aid patients has become poorer _____ Maj   Min   No   DK

e) Other aspects of audiology departments work have suffered due to concentration on DR_____ Maj   Min   No   DK

Part III

Summary of Main Findings

36 DR Pilot Projects: Summary of Main Findings

1. Direct Referral (DR) systems for hearing aid provision were set up at 12 NHS Hearing Aid Centres based in hospitals around England. Termed 'Pilot' schemes, these were evaluated and compared with the Traditional Referral system (TR). Pilot Centres were requested to consider building two special elements into their DR schemes: community provision, and involvement of the private sector. Six included some element of community provision, and four engaged the involvement of private dispensers. (Section 4.2).

2. Waiting times from GP referral to fitting of the hearing aid were substantially reduced under the DR systems. All 12 Centres experienced at least some degree of reduction. Overall, the median wait during the latter part of the pilot period was 28 weeks for TR patients, compared to 11 weeks for DRs. The reduction in waiting times was mainly due to the fact that DR patients avoided the wait for an ENT clinic appointment. The average waiting times at 16 'pre-existing' DR schemes were similar in length: 26 weeks for TRs, and 13 weeks for DRs. (Sections 6.3 and 32.1).

3. Under a DR system, technicians cross-refer to ENT any patients they consider to need a medical opinion. The numbers of cross-referrals during the pilot period varied considerably from one Centre to another. The lowest rate at any Centre was 3%, and the highest 44%, with an overall proportion of 18%. In 69% of cross-referral cases the ENT doctor decided that no further action was required. (Sections 7.3 and 9.5).

4. During the pilot period, all DR patients received a safety-check by a local ENT doctor. The examinations made by technicians (including private dispensers) were compared with the ENT checks on the same patients for a total sample of over 2,300. Technicians were considered to have failed in their management of the patient in 2.2% of cases. However, many of these instances were rated as being not serious or of only moderate severity. The rate of potentially serious technician management failures was 0.64%, or about 1 in every 156 patients. The rate for NHS technicians alone was 0.56%, or about 1 in every 177. Direct Referral is invariably run in conjunction with a TR service, and it is estimated that the number of additional potentially serious failures that can be expected across both systems as a result of introducing DR is around 1 in every 430 patients (Sections 9.7 to 9.8).

5. Two external specialists were employed who conducted independent medical examinations of samples of 239 DR and 216 TR patients across 9 of the pilot Centres. Two experts in audiological medicine, each working independently, then compared the results of these examinations with the previous examinations made by technicians and local ENT doctors. On the basis of the specialist examinations and expert assessments, around 5% of all DR patients were found to attend with conditions considered by the experts to have potentially serious consequences for the patient, compared to 10% of TR patients. (Section 10.6).

6. Technicians were assessed by the experts as having made potentially serious failures of management in 2.3% of the DR cases, and to have picked up 54% of all DR patients with potentially serious conditions. The local ENT doctors who also saw these patients (excepting a few missing cases) were judged to have made 3.0% potentially serious failures and to have correctly managed 26% of all potentially serious conditions. However, there was evidence that the safety-checks of DR patients were done to a less stringent standard than normal ENT examinations; and amongst the TR sample ENT doctors were judged to have appropriately managed 41% of potentially serious cases. It is important to note that technician management and doctor management are not equivalent things, as the doctor has to make more complex decisions than the technician, and the two cannot be directly compared. (Section 10.8).

7. The principal reason for the sizable numbers of apparent 'failures' of management appears to be a difference in attitude between the experts (and specialists) and many local doctors with regard to the right way to manage instances of asymmetrical loss – an indicator of possible acoustic neuroma. 70% of the cases rated by the experts as potentially serious doctor failures were of this kind. Local doctors tended not to undertake further management in such cases, the general opinion appearing to be that in elderly patients an operation may do more harm than good. The experts and specialists, however, considered intervention to be advisable in many of these cases. Over half of the technician failures were also of this form, probably because technicians were working to the practices of their local doctors. It is of interest to note that these cases failed the TTSA guidelines on asymmetry. (Section 10.11).

8. The failure rate for DR as a system is higher than for technicians alone, because even if a technician appropriately cross-refers a patient, there is a chance that the examining doctor will fail in his management. In terms of raw counts, the number of patients with potentially serious conditions that went undetected was a little lower under DR than TR. However, the rate of potentially serious pathology was substantially lower amongst the DR sample to begin with, and in terms of detecting pathology when present, the TR system fared better. According to the experts, on average 41% of all potentially serious cases were correctly managed under TR, as against 24% under DR. The difference was not statistically significant, but the samples were small. (Section 10.9).

9. As a rule, Centres operating a DR system do so in combination with TR. It was estimated that with the proportional mix of DR and TR patients found towards the end of the pilot schemes, around 36% of all potentially serious cases (i.e. DR and TR) would be correctly managed. This compares to 41% under TR operating on its own. Thus, the introduction of DR increases the overall risk to patients - that is, the probability of a potentially serious condition remaining undetected – by about 5% (with an approximate 95% confidence interval of plus or minus 4%). Expressed in terms of a rate over all patients seen, the difference amounts to about 1 additional potentially serious management failure out of every 300 patients seen. This rate is quite close to the estimate of 1 in 430 obtained from the comparison of technician and ENT examinations on all DR patients coming through the schemes (see 4, above). (Section 10.10).

10. The increased risk associated with the introduction of DR needs to be seen in the context of several mitigating factors. Firstly, these are *potentially* serious cases – a number of which may prove to be not serious at all. Secondly, any missed conditions might be picked up at subsequent visits by the patient to their GP. Thirdly, an increased risk of 5% is in fact much smaller than the variation that already exists between ENT doctors (i.e. smaller than the possible increase in risk due to being seen by one doctor rather than another). Fourthly, DR removes substantial numbers of patients from the ENT queue, allowing other patients (who themselves might have serious conditions) to be seen more quickly. And finally, under many TR systems patients referred for hearing aids are selected out and seen by quite junior ENT doctors. A DR system run by experienced technicians where cross-referrals are examined by senior doctors might prove safer than this arrangement. (Section 10.11).

11. Given that there is a potential for increased risk under DR, it is worth considering a number of steps which can be taken to reduce the risk further. (1) GPs need to be encouraged to do a better job of selecting appropriate patients for Direct Referral, and of dewaxing patients prior to referral. (2) It is recommended that only highly experienced technicians should be allowed to screen DR patients, and that any cross-referrals are seen only by ENT doctors with high levels of experience. (3) Technicians need clear and precise criteria to follow, particularly with regard to asymmetrical loss, and they must ensure that they follow these. (4) It is suggested that the ENT community address the general issue of how best to manage elderly patients exhibiting asymmetrical hearing loss. (Section 10.11).

12. Patient satisfaction with the DR schemes was very high. At all pilot Centres DR patients expressed higher levels of satisfaction with the service received than did TR patients. Overall, 84% of DR patients made very positive statements about the service, compared to 59% of TR patients. DR patients were also more satisfied with the time they had waited for their first appointment: 55% of DRs were positive as against 14% of TRs. (Section 11.4).

13. At all but one pilot Centre DR patients were more likely to be seen on time at the first appointment. In all, 91% were seen within 10 minutes of appointment time, compared to 55% of TRs; and 4% queued for a half-hour or more as against 30%. (Section 11.1).

14. The majority of both TR and DR patients go through the provision process in just two appointments (not including the initial visit to the GP or any follow-ups). The number needing more appointments varied considerably from place to place. At seven projects more DRs than TRs had extra appointments, and at just two the reverse occurred. For Centres where comparable data was available, the overall percentage of TRs having more than two appointments was 24%, and for DRs it was 42%. Also, slightly more of the DR group experienced 4 or more appointments. (Section 11.2).

15. Despite the above, DR patients on the whole spent less time keeping appointments (time travelling and at appointments). This was the case at 6 out of 9 Centres for which figures could be computed. DRs spent an average of 3 hours 17 mins on appointments, while TRs spent 4 hours 4 mins. Most of the difference was due to DR patients being seen more promptly at the first appointment. (Section 11.3).

16. Technician satisfaction with the DR systems was very high. Large majorities reported that job satisfaction, job interest, and variety were better than before DR. Smaller majorities felt the same about the level of responsibility involved and the personal involvement with patients. In no instance did more than one technician feel that any of these things had become worse. However, notable minorities felt that levels of workload and stress were worse. Twenty-two out of twenty-six technicians wanted to continue to see DR patients after the end of the pilot period. The other four were uncertain, two because of increased workload, and two because of high numbers of poor quality referrals from GPs. (Section 12.2).

17. Presented with a list of possible benefits of their DR scheme, head technicians rated the following most highly: a better quality of service (rated 'major benefit' by 10 out of 12); a faster service (8 out of 12); integrates the whole process of provision (8 out of 12). These were also the most highly rated items in the survey of pre-existing schemes. (Sections 13.2 and 33.6).

18. Consultants, from a different list, considered 'a faster service to hearing aid patients' to be the single most important benefit (rated 'Major' by 9 out of 10). Consultants in the pre-existing schemes also rated this the most important benefit. Another notable benefit for both sets of consultants was that DR frees up ENT time for more serious cases. (Sections 13.2 and 33.7).

19. Head technicians rated a list of possible problems they may have experienced. Very few 'major problem' ratings were given, but three items stood out as being the most important: number of DR patients being cross-referred to ENT; quality of referrals from GPs; and number of DRs needing a dewax. On the whole, problems had declined since the start of the

pilots, and problems at the pre- existing schemes – which had been running longer – were lower again. (Sections 13.4 and 33.2).

20. Consultants at the pilot schemes found the numbers being cross-referred to ENT to be the biggest problem (1 major and 4 minor). No other item got any 'major' ratings. However, the biggest problem at the pre-existing schemes was lack of technicians, followed by the numbers of DR patients requiring wax removal. (Sections 13.5 and 33.4).

21. For both TR and DR, direct costs of staff time and materials (including the aid) were computed for the GP, Hearing Aid Centre, and ENT. On the whole, there was very little cost difference: less than £1 (in favour of TR) out of a total cost of around £59 on average. Under slightly different assumptions, the cost difference disappears completely. The differences between Centres in terms of cost were not very large, but in the main, at Centres with low numbers of cross-referrals DR tended to be a little cheaper, but where cross-referral rates were high TR proved a slightly more economical service. Even at high rates of cross-referral however, the cost difference is no more than a few pounds. (Section 15.2).

22. There was just one Centre where DR patients were seen in the community who would otherwise have come to the main site. The average additional cost to this Centre of serving a patient in the community was estimated to be £11.43 per patient. (Section 15.4).

23. A total of four private dispensers were involved, each at a different Centre. Two dispensers demonstrated much lower rates of cross-referral (both statistically significant) compared to NHS technicians at the same Centre, and a third was lower but not significantly so. These lower rates may suggest that dispensers were not cross-referring all patients they should have. The work of two dispensers in particular was found to be poor in other respects as well. (Section 18).

24. The numbers of referrals made by GPs that were inappropriate were generally high. The estimated rates vary between 19% and 60%, and although these figures are approximate, they are close to other, published, findings. It was also estimated that around one-quarter of all patients with potentially serious conditions were coming through DR (with the rest through TR). All the evidence indicates that many GPs are poor at selecting patients for DR. Furthermore, the rates of inappropriate referrals did not decline between the first and second halves of the projects. It is clear from this that for Direct Referral to be successful, it must rely on the abilities of technicians to detect serious pathology as much as on GPs. (Section 17.3).

25. At 11 of the 12 Centres both head technicians and consultants were happy with the way that the pilots had gone, and satisfied with service quality and safety. All of these 11 Centres continued Direct Referral after the end of the pilot period. The remaining Centre had not found that DR held any substantive benefits over their TR system. They were also concerned

about the large numbers of poor quality GP referrals, and the safety of the procedure. This Centre halted the Direct Referral service. Just 2 of the pre-existing DR schemes have been halted permanently; one because of staff shortages, and the other because of large numbers of poor quality referrals. (Sections 14.1 to 14.3, and section 28.1).

37 Survey of Pre-Existing Schemes: Summary of Main Findings

1. A postal survey of all 158 Hearing Aid Centres in England was conducted in February – April 1991. A total of 144 returns were received (91% response rate). Of these, 56 (39%) operate or had operated a Direct Referral scheme (DR). (Section 25).

2. Twenty-one Centres with experience of DR were selected for interviewing. These Centres represented as broad a range of types as possible, and included all those that had stopped or temporarily suspended DR. The head technician was interviewed at each of the 21 Centres, and at 16 an ENT consultant was also interviewed, or (in 4 cases) completed a postal questionnaire. (Section 26).

3. The most common reason – by far – given for the introduction of Direct referral was that it was in order to reduce ENT waiting lists. This was often coupled with the related aim of freeing up ENT time for more serious cases. (Section 27).

4. Four Centres had temporarily suspended Direct Referral at some period, whilst another two had stopped completely. In all cases of suspension, lack of audiological technicians was the major reason. Of the two Centres that had stopped completely, staff shortage resulting in very long waiting lists was the main cause at one, while the poor quality of referrals from GPs was the major reason at the other. Safety of the procedure was not an issue in suspending or stopping any of the schemes. (Section 28).

5. Consultants showed high levels of confidence in the screening abilities of their technicians. However, only one Centre is known to have formally evaluated the safety of the procedure. The result of this evaluation was that the consultants were happy with the safety of the scheme and decided to implement it permanently. (Sections 30.3 and 30.4).

6. There was much variety of opinion, both between and within Centres, as to who was medically responsible for directly referred patients. Only one Centre (the same as in point 5 above) had formally addressed the issue. However, in none of the 21 Centres had litigation relating to Direct Referral ever occurred. (Section 31).

7. Typical waiting times from GP referral to fitting of the aid for both DR and for the traditional referral system (TR) running in parallel were available for 16 Centres. Under TR, typical waiting times ranged from 12 weeks up to 63 weeks with 9 Centres having typical waits of 6 months or more. Under DR, the range was 4 weeks to 68 weeks. However, the latter figure is exceptional, as only 2 Centres had typical waits of 6 months or more. Overall, the waiting time for DR was half of the wait for TR: 13 weeks compared to 26 weeks. In only 2 of the 16 Centres was the waiting time under DR longer than under TR. In both these Centres the DR waiting list had grown as a result of reductions in the number of technicians. This shows that the continuance of shorter waiting times depends upon adequate staffing levels being maintained in the Hearing Aid Centre. (Section 32).

8. The shorter waiting times for DR compared to TR could nearly all be accounted for by the fact that patients were not having to wait for an ENT clinic appointment. Overall, the times between ear examination and fitting of the aid were very similar for both systems. (Section 32).

9. Presented with a list of possible problems they may have experienced with their DR scheme, head technicians identified the following as the most important: general workload (31% 'major problem'); funding (27%); number of patients needing a dewax (25%); number of direct referrals (19%) and lack of staff (18%). (Section 33.2).

10. Regarding the important issue of quality of referrals from GPs, in 35% of the Centres there was some degree of problem, although only one Centre rated this as major. The percentage of Centres stating that referral quality had been a problem in the past, however, was much higher: 69%. The major complaint was patients attending with wax, which the GPs should have removed. A few staff expressed the opinion that some GPs intentionally abused the system to bypass ENT waiting lists. (Sections 33.2 and 33.3).

11. Twenty head technicians had experienced 'no problem' with patient satisfaction under DR. The 'minor problem' at the remaining Centre was due to long waiting times. Some were of the opinion that DR patients were more satisfied with their service than TR patients. (Section 33.2).

12. Consultants were also presented with a list of possible problems, from the ENT point of view. They identified the following as most important: lack of technicians (30% 'major problem'); and DR patients being sent to ENT for dewax (15%). (Section 33.4).

13. None of the consultants had found any problems with the competence of technicians. (Section 33.4).

14. Shortage of technicians appears to be a national problem, firstly in that a number of Centres do not have the budget to employ the optimum number of technicians for the population served. Secondly, there is a shortage of people

wanting to be trained as technicians and therefore when jobs do become available, frequently the posts cannot be filled. (Section 33.2).

15. Presented with a list of possible benefits, head technicians rated the following most highly: a faster service for patients (75% 'major benefit'); a better quality service to patients (72%); integration of the whole process of provision (74%); Direct Referral makes the technician's job more varied and interesting (75%); technicians feel more valued and respected (65%); and DR provides a more personal service to patients as individuals (63%). (Section 33.6).

16. From the ENT point of view, consultants viewed the most important benefits as: a faster service to hearing aid patients (rated major by 93%); the freeing of ENT time for more serious cases (62%); and the development of a more professional attitude to their work by technicians (58%). (Section 33.7).

17. With regard to the disadvantages of DR, technicians rated only one of these substantially. This was the extra paperwork generated by Direct Referral (a major disadvantage to 22% and a minor disadvantage to 50%). Another disadvantage mentioned by a couple of technicians was that some consultants pass patients with hearing problems across to them when they should really be seen in ENT. (Section 33.8).

18. Consultants rated only one disadvantage as important: that as a result of Direct Referral ENT doctors have become distanced from the hearing aid side of ENT work (15% 'major disadvantage' and 46% 'minor disadvantage'). This is a factor which needs to be considered carefully by the ENT and Audiology communities, as it is possible that widespread adoption of DR systems could eventually result in a lack of ENT doctors skilled in this aspect of the field. (Section 33.9).

19. Almost all of the technicians (20 out of 21) were enthusiastic about their DR system. The one technician who did not express enthusiasm had suffered from staffing and organisational problems, but felt that in theory DR was a good idea. (Section 34.1).

20. The great majority of consultants (9 out of 13 asked directly) also believed DR was a good idea. Three others felt that the benefits of DR could outweigh the disadvantages, subject to certain conditions. Only one consultant expressed a negative opinion. This was based this upon personal experience of 2 Direct Referral schemes, one of which was causing problems although the other was running satisfactorily. (Section 34.2).

38 Some Pointers for Centres Thinking of Implementing a Direct Referral System

1. ENT consultants or audiological physicians should ensure that technicians who will be screening DR patients are familiar with all the important forms of pathology they are likely to encounter. It is also recommended that ENT audit a proportion of the patients seen by technicians, at least during the early months of a new DR system.

2. Centres will also need to establish a set of guidelines for technicians to help them identify DR patients who need to be passed across to an ENT doctor. Most Centres find the guidelines drawn up by the TTSA (appendix I.III) a useful basis, with perhaps some minor modifications or additions. It is relevant to note that under the pilot schemes over one-third of all technician management failures, and *nearly two-thirds of serious failures*, were cases of asymmetrical loss that were not cross-referred but which the local ENT doctor felt needed investigation or review. It would seem very important, therefore, that consultants pay particular attention to the criteria they set regarding asymmetry, ensure that the rules are unambiguous, and that technicians follow them correctly.

3. GPs should also be provided with precise criteria for selecting patients for Direct Referral. It seems advisable to keep the criteria list short and simple, as many GPs may not adhere to a complex list. An example list appears in appendix I.VII of this report. Some of the pilot Centres had a problem with patients coming through the system who already had hearing aids, and therefore the example list has been designed to alleviate this.

4. It is advised that an age criterion for DR patients of at least 60 years is adopted. Given that under the pilot projects technicians did miss a small number of potentially serious conditions, it would be prudent to ensure that all under-60's are examined by an ENT doctor.

5. 'Open Days', seminars, or presentations for GPs explaining the scheme and referral criteria are a good idea. However, a common experience is that such events are often very poorly attended, and therefore it is important to do all you can to encourage attendance.

6. Take-up of the DR scheme by GPs is quite likely to be slow at first. Even so, it may be a good idea to start in a small way – say with a few selected GP

practices – so that any teething problems can be sorted before the service is made more widely available.

7. A proportion of DR patients will attend with significant ear pathology. Given this, it is advisable that all DR patients are seen by *senior* technicians with several years experience.

8. When booking DR patients in, time will need to be allotted for the technician to take the history, examine the patient, and complete any paperwork. It is suggested that, at least initially, 30 minutes is allowed for these tasks (or a full hour for these plus testing and impressions). Once familiarity with the procedures has been established the allotted time can probably be reduced.

9. If possible, it may be a good idea to arrange things such that each patient is seen by the same technician at every stage of the process. Both patients and technicians seem to prefer this, and it may possibly have benefits in terms of post-fitting rehabilitation.

10. It is likely that a significant proportion of the referrals will be inappropriate and many of these will need to be cross-referred to ENT. It is necessary to ensure that suitable arrangements for the handling of cross-referrals have been agreed with ENT prior to implementing the scheme.

11. It is also likely that in most cases of cross-referral ENT will decide that no additional action is required. This was the case in some 70% of cross-referrals during the pilot schemes.

12. Where a cross-referred DR patient will not be seen by ENT until some future date, a decision needs to be made whether or not to go ahead and fit a hearing aid (assuming one is appropriate) in the meantime. The drawback to proceeding with fitting is that a substantial proportion of patients, once they have got their aid, refuse to come back for the ENT appointment. This could lead to some cases of serious pathology going untreated.

13. In order to ensure that safety-levels for DR patients are as far as possible kept on a par with those for TR patients, it is recommended that all DR patients cross-referred by technicians are seen by a senior ENT doctor, and that the doctor is informed of the reasons for cross-referral.

14. Communication with referring GPs is essential if referral quality is going to improve. Where patients are crossed immediately to ENT, it is a good idea to write to the GP explaining the reasons for cross-referring and those elements (if any) of the criteria list he/she failed to follow. If possible, provide GPs with a 'hot-line' telephone number that they can ring for advice about the scheme if they need it.

15. It has been found that the great majority of GPs only directly refer two or three patients in a year. Therefore the overall quality of referrals is unlikely to improve very much over the first year of operation.

16. A number of patients will attend with significant amounts of wax, no matter how strongly GPs are urged to remove wax before referring. A mechanism for dealing with patients needing wax removal should be worked out before implementing the DR scheme. The most common are either:
a) ensure that the DR clinics are held when an ENT doctor/staff nurse is available to dewax; or b) send such patients back to their GP for dewax.

17. Where the presence of wax prevents clear examination of an ear-drum, it is recommended that the patient is either be re-examined after wax removal or cross-referred to ENT. It is unsafe to just assume that the drum is o.k.

18. It is essential to ensure that technicians have legal cover for their work with DR patients. Probably the best way to do this is to arrange for DR work to be part of the technicians' job description, which ensures that the Health Authority, Trust, or other employing body will accept liability for their actions. (See Chapter 23).

19. It is easy to underestimate the amount of additional clerical and paperwork a DR system generates for the Hearing Aid Centre. It is advisable to have a designated clerk to take charge of this work, otherwise it can consume a great deal of technician time.

20. A charge will need to set for fund-holding GPs / Health Authorities using the DR system. In calculating this it should be borne in mind that the full economic cost may exceed that of other Hearing Aid Centre appointments. This is because a significant proportion of DR patients will need to be cross-referred to ENT. Some Centres which have not allowed for this in the charge require GPs to re-refer such patients to ENT, so that the cost of the ENT appointment is not lost. This arrangement has the benefit that it discourages GPs from sending inappropriate patients via DR, but is less efficient than cross-referring straight to ENT, and can delay patient treatment.

21. It may be that the introduction of DR will increase the demand for hearing aids. This will have implications for Hearing Aid Centre expenditure, though it is unlikely that much effect on demand will be noticed during the first year. Any increase in numbers of fittings is going to have financial repercussions for a long time, because the new users will be making demands on post-fitting services for many years.

References

Baguley D. M., Harries M. L., and Moffat D. A. (1989) Direct Referral for Hearing Aids: Problems and Pitfalls. Unpublished manuscript.

Bamford J. (1988) TTSA Guidelines for Hearing Aid Direct Referrals. British Association of Audiological Scientists. *Newsletter*, 13: 16–17.

Bellini M. J., Beesley P., Perrett C. and Pickles J. M. (1989) Hearing-aids: Can they be Safely Prescribed without Medical Supervision? An Analysis of Patients Referred for Hearing-aids. *Clinical Otolaryngology*, 14: 415–418.

Brookes D. N. (1990) Hearing Aid Fitting Costs in the NHS. *British Journal of Audiology* 24: 357–358 (letter).

Campbell J. B., Nigam A., and Bland N. C. (1989) Provision of Hearing Aids: Does Specialist Assessment Cause Delay? *British Medical Journal*, 299: 855–856 (letter).

Griffin J. (1988) Drug Induced Ototoxicity. *British Journal of Audiology*, 22, 195–210.

Harries M. L. L., Baguley D. M. and Moffat D. A. (1989) Hearing Aids – A Case for Review. *Journal of Laryngology and Otology*, 103: 850–852.

Hartmann D. P. (1977) Considerations in the choice of interobserver reliability estimates. *Journal of Applied Behaviour Analysis*, 10, 103–116.

Hawthorne M. R., Desmond A. N., Clarke G. P. and Robertshaw D. (1991) Direct Referral Hearing Aid Provision in the Over Sixties Age Group. *The Journal of Laryngology and Otology*, 105: 825–827.

Johnsson L. and Hawkins J. (1972) Sensory and Neural Degeneration With Aging as seen in Microdissections of the Human Inner Ear. *Annals of Otology, Rhinology, and Laryngology*, 81, 179–193.

Lim D. P. and Stephens S. D. G. (1991) Clinical Investigation of Hearing Loss in the Elderly. *Clinical Otolaryngology*, 16, 288–293.

Makishima K. (1978) Arteriolar Sclerosis as a Cause of Presbyacucis. *Archives of Otolaryngology*, 93, 161–166.

Prinsley P., Premachandra D. J., and Madden G. (1989) Dispensing Hearing Aids in the Community. *The Lancet*, August 26th, 500–501 (letter).

Royal National Institute for the Deaf (1984) *A Survey of National Health Service Hearing Aid Services*. London.

Royal National Institute for the Deaf (1988) *Hearing Aids – the Case for Change*. London.

Royal National Institute for the Deaf (1989) *Hearing Aids – the Developing Debate*. London.

Stephens S. D. G. (1983) Rehabilitation and Service Needs. In *Hearing Science and Hearing Disorders* Latman M. E. and Haggard M. P. (Eds). Academic Press, London, 283 – 324.

Stephens S. D. G. (1992) Personal Communication.

Ward P. R. (1980) Treatment of Elderly Adults with Impaired Hearing: Resources, Outcome and Efficiency. *Journal of Epidemiology and Community Health* 34: 65–68.

Watson C. and Crowther J. A. (1989) Provision of Hearing Aids: Does Specialist Assessment Cause Delay? *British Medical Journal*, 299: 437–439.

Printed in the United Kingdom for HMSO
Dd297625 3/94 C20 G3397 10170